Environmental Health

Environmental Health

Dade W. Moeller

Harvard University Press
Cambridge, Massachusetts
London, England
1992

Copyright © 1992 by the President and Fellows of Harvard College
All rights reserved
Printed in the United States of America
10 9 8 7 6 5 4 3 2 1

This book is printed on acid-free paper.

Library of Congress Cataloging-in-Publication Data
Moeller, D. W. (Dade W.)
    Environmental health
  Dade W. Moeller.
        p.   cm.
    Includes index.
    ISBN 0-674-25858-4 (alk. paper)
    1. Environmental health.   I. Title.
    [DNLM: 1. Environmental Health.   2. Environmental Pollution.   WA
30 M693e]
  RA565.M64   1992
  616.9'8—dc20
  DNLM/DLC
  for Library of Congress   91-20836
                                        CIP

To Betty Jean, who has been the joy of my life for more than forty years, and to Rad, Mark, Kehne, Matt, and Anne, who never cease to make us proud

Contents

Preface

This book is an outgrowth of a survey course, "Principles of Environmental Health," that I have taught at the Harvard School of Public Health for the past twenty-five years and, in modified form, at the Harvard University Extension School.

Although the literature abounds with monographs on particular aspects of environmental health (air pollution, water pollution, solid waste disposal, and so on), and although more and more courses are being offered on the subject, there are few textbooks that provide comprehensive coverage of the field. In this book I present topics from both local and global perspectives, and in relation to both short- and long-range impacts. In my review of individual segments of the environment—such as air, water, and food—I highlight the necessity to consider the interrelationships of these and other segments in the development and application of controls. I also examine health hazards in the workplace; the control of insects and rodents; the disposal of solid, radioactive, and hazardous wastes; the effects, uses, and management of ionizing and nonionizing radiation; accidents as a cause of injuries and deaths; environmental monitoring; risk assessment as applied to the development of environmental standards; response preparedness for natural and man-made disasters; and the occupational and environmental impacts of energy use. Often in my general coverage of various aspects of environmental health I use examples pertaining to ionizing radiation to illustrate important concepts. I do so not only because this is my area of expertise, but also because approaches to controlling occupational and environmental health problems associated with ionizing radiation are, in some respects, more advanced than the approaches used in other fields of environmental health.

As would be expected for an undertaking of this magnitude, I am grateful to a host of fellow environmental and public health professionals for sharing their talents and expertise with me. Special thanks to my colleagues at the Harvard School of Public Health, William A. Burgess, Melvin W. First, Peter Goldman, David Hemenway, John B. Little, Jacob Shapiro, R. Jeremy Sherwood, and Andrew Spielman. Other associates who provided invaluable support include Gerard Bertrand, Douglas J. Crawford-Brown, Thomas S. Crowther, Paul M. Newberne, Cynthia Palmer, Howard Peters, Floyd B. Taylor, Julian A. Waller, and Ellen Wasserman. I also thank Harvey V. Fineberg, Dean of the Harvard School of Public Health, for his support and encouragement. Finally, I deeply appreciate the editorial suggestions of Ann Hawthorne at Harvard University Press.

And God pronounced a blessing upon Noah and his sons and said to them, be fruitful and multiply and fill the earth.

And the fear of you and the dread and terror of you shall be upon every beast of the land, every bird of the air, all that creeps upon the ground, and upon all the fishes of the sea. Into your hands they are delivered.

Genesis 9:1–2

Abbreviations

AAEE	American Academy of Environmental Engineers
ACGIH	American Conference of Governmental Industrial Hygienists
AMA	American Medical Association
ASME	American Society of Mechanical Engineers
BEIR	Committee on the Biological Effects of Ionizing Radiation, National Research Council
BRWM	Board on Radioactive Waste Management, National Research Council
CDC	Centers for Disease Control, U.S. Department of Health and Human Services
DOE	U.S. Department of Energy
EPA	U.S. Environmental Protection Agency
EPRI	Electric Power Research Institute
FEMA	Federal Emergency Management Agency
ICRP	International Commission on Radiological Protection
IRPA	International Radiation Protection Association
NCRP	National Council on Radiation Protection and Measurements
NRC	U.S. Nuclear Regulatory Commission
OSHA	Occupational Safety and Health Administration
UNESCO	United Nations Educational, Scientific, and Cultural Organization

1

The Scope of Environmental Health

Many aspects of human well-being are influenced by the environment, and many diseases can be initiated, sustained, or exacerbated by environmental factors. For that reason, understanding and controlling people's interactions with their environment is an important component of public health. In its broadest sense, environmental health is the subfield of public health concerned with assessing and controlling the impacts of people on their environment (including vegetation, other animals, and natural and historic landmarks) and the impacts of the environment on them.

The field of environmental health is defined more by the problems faced than by the specific approaches used. These problems include the treatment and disposal of liquid and airborne wastes, the elimination or reduction of stresses in the workplace, purification of drinking-water supplies, the impacts of overpopulation and inadequate or unsafe food supplies, and the development and use of measures to protect hospital and other medical workers from being infected with diseases such as acquired immune deficiency syndrome (AIDS). Environmental health professionals also face long-range problems, including the effects of toxic chemicals and radioactive waste, acidic deposition, depletion of the ozone layer, and global warming. The complexity of these issues requires multidisciplinary approaches for their evaluation and control. A team coping with a major environmental health problem may include scientists, physicians, epidemiologists, engineers, economists, lawyers, mathematicians, and managers. Input from all these experts is essential to the development and success of broad strategies that take into account both lifestyles and the environment.

The Systems Approach

One of the major goals of environmental health professionals is to understand the various ways in which humans interact with their environment. Comprehensive and accurate evaluations require an integrated "systems approach" that assesses an environmental problem in its entirety. At least four steps are involved:

1. Determine the source and nature of each environmental contaminant or stress.
2. Assess how and in what form it comes into contact with people.
3. Measure the effects.
4. Apply controls when and where appropriate.

Instead of focusing on a single pollutant facility by facility, environmental health professionals gather data on all the discharges from a given facility, as well as all the sources of a given pollutant and all the pollutants being deposited in a region, regardless of their nature, origin, or pathway (Train, 1990).

While tracing the source of a contaminant and its pathways, environmental health professionals conduct studies to determine its effects on human health. Working with biologists, toxicologists, respiratory physiologists, epidemiologists, and other public health personnel, they establish to the extent possible quantitative relationships between the exposure or dose and its effects. On the basis of these data, they set acceptable limits for exposures to the contaminant or stress.

To assess the effects of exposures correctly, environmental health workers must take into account not only the fact that exposures may derive from multiple sources and enter the body by several routes, but also the fact that elements in the environment are constantly interacting, so that in the course of transport or degradation, agents that were originally not toxic to people may become so, and vice versa. If the concentration of a contaminant is relatively uniform (for example, a substance in the air), local or regional sampling may provide adequate data to estimate human exposures. If concentrations vary considerably over space and time and the people being exposed move about extensively, it may be necessary to measure exposures to individual workers or members of the public by providing them with small, lightweight, battery-operated portable monitoring units. Development of such monitors and the specifications for their use requires the expertise of air pollution engineers, industrial hygienists, chemists and chemical engineers, electronics experts, and quality-control personnel. Once the levels of exposure are known, these can be compared with existing standards, and controls can be applied when and where warranted.

Defining the Environment

To do their work effectively, environmental health professionals must keep in mind that there are many ways of defining the environment. One approach, used in Chapter 2, considers the indoor versus the outdoor (ambient) environment. Another, used in Chapter 3, narrows the focus to the workplace. Although every definition has deficiencies, each offers a different perspective that can broaden understanding of the complexities involved in potential threats to environmental health. Consideration of the full range of existing environments is also necessary if a systems approach is to be used in controlling associated problems.

The Inner versus Outer Environment

From the standpoint of the human body, there are two environments, the one inside and the one outside. Separating these environments are three principal barriers: the skin, which protects the body from contaminants outside it; the gastrointestinal (GI) tract, which protects the inner body from contaminants that have been ingested; and the lungs, which protect the inner body from contaminants that have been inhaled (Table 1.1). Each of these barriers is vulnerable under certain conditions. Contaminants can penetrate to the inner body through the skin by dissolving the layer of wax provided by the sebaceous glands. Airborne materials of respirable size can be deposited in the lungs and, if they are soluble, absorbed. Soluble compounds that make their way into the GI tract can be readily absorbed and taken into the cells. The lungs are by far the most fragile and susceptible barrier. An average adult breathes about 800 cubic feet (20 cubic meters), or more than 50 pounds (24 kg), of air per day. Because people cannot be selective about the air that is available, the lungs are considered to be the most important pathway for the intake of environmental contaminants.

Table 1.1   Characteristics of the principal barriers between the outer and inner body

Barrier	Area ft^2	Area m^2	Thickness in.	Thickness μm	Weight lbs	Weight kg	Daily exposure lbs	Daily exposure kg
Skin	21	2	4×10^{-3}	100	30	12–16	Variable	
GI tract	2,150	200	4×10^{-4}	10–12	15	7	4–6	2–3
Lungs	1,500	140	1×10^{-5}	0.2–0.4	2	0.8–0.9	50	24

Fortunately, the body also has protective mechanisms to deal with many contaminants that do penetrate its barriers. For the GI tract, these include vomiting through the mouth or rapid excretion through the bowels (as in the case of diarrhea). Similarly, materials entering the circulatory system can be detoxified in the liver or excreted through the kidneys. Mechanisms for protecting the lungs range from simple coughing to cleansing by macrophages that engulf and promote the removal of foreign materials.

The Personal versus Ambient Environment

Another definition contrasts the "personal" environment, over which people have control, with the working or ambient environment, over which they may have essentially no control. Although people commonly think of the working or ambient environment as posing the greater threat, environmental health experts estimate that the personal environment, shaped by hygiene, diet, sexual practices, exercise, use of drugs and alcohol, and frequency of medical checkups, often has much more influence on well-being. Table 1.2 summarizes the estimated contributions of these various factors. According to public health experts, the personal environment may contribute to 75 percent or more of cancer deaths in the general U.S. population (Doll and Peto, 1981). Smoking plays the largest single role, accounting for more than one in every six deaths in the United States (Surgeon General, 1989). The amount of pollution taken into a smoker's lungs as a result of inhaling the various products from cigarettes is several orders of magnitude greater than the amount normally inhaled as a result of industrial airborne pollution.

The Solid, Liquid, and Gaseous Environments

The environment can also be considered as existing in one of three forms—gaseous, liquid, or solid. Each of these is subject to pollution, and people interact with all of them (Figure 1.1). Examples include releases of particulates and gases into the atmosphere; the discharge of wastes into water; and the disposal of solid waste, particularly plastics and toxic chemicals. Often attempts to control pollution in one form can create pollution in another. For example, the incineration of solid waste causes atmospheric pollution; the use of scrubbers and other types of air-cleaning systems can produce large amounts of solid waste; chemical treatment of liquid waste can produce large quantities of sludge; and sulfur and nitrogen oxides discharged into the atmosphere can be brought down to the earth in the form of acidic deposition. Such shifts or transfers can have significant effects; for example, wastewater treatment plants in Philadelphia are estimated to generate 25 percent of that region's airborne toxic organic pollutants (Hahn and Males, 1990).

Clearly, what is done to the environment in one form will almost certainly affect it in others. A systems approach ensures that each

Table 1.2   Proportion of cancer deaths attributable to various factors

Factor	% of all cancer deaths	
	Best estimate	Range of acceptable estimates
Diet	35	10–70
Tobacco	30	25–40
Reproductive and sexual behavior	7	1–13
Occupation	4	2–8
Alcohol consumption	3	2–4
Geophysical factors	3	2–4
Infections	10?	1–?
Medicines and medical procedures	1	0.5–3
Food additives, pollution, and industrial products	< 4	< 2–7

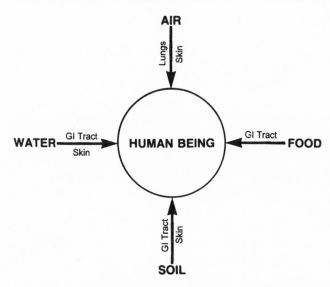

Figure 1.1 Routes of human exposure through the solid, liquid, and gaseous environments

problem is examined not in isolation but in terms of how it interacts with and can affect other segments of the environment and people's daily lives.

The Chemical, Biological, Physical, and Socioeconomic Environments

Another perspective considers the environment in terms of the four avenues or mechanisms by which various factors affect people's health. Thus, *chemical* constituents and contaminants include toxic waste and pesticides in the general environment, chemicals used in the home and in industrial operations, and preservatives used in foods. *Biological* contaminants include various disease organisms that may be present in food and water, those that can be transmitted by insects and animals, and those that can be transmitted by person-to-person contact. *Physical* factors that influence health and well-being range from workplace or traffic accidents, to excessive noise, heat, and cold, to ionizing and nonionizing radiation. Though perhaps more difficult to measure than the others, *socioeconomic* factors significantly

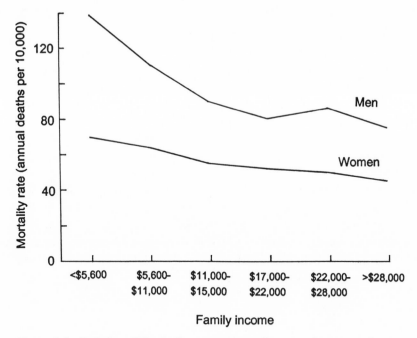

Figure 1.2   Relation of family income to mortality rates for men and women,
United States, 1980

affect people's lives and health (Figure 1.2). People who live in economically depressed neighborhoods are less healthy than those who
live in more affluent ones. The factors contributing to these differences range from inadequate nutrition and medical care to stressful
social conditions.

Addressing Environmental Health Problems

In contrast to physicians, who traditionally deal with one patient at a
time, environmental health specialists must consider entire populations. To the extent possible, they must also try to anticipate problems
in order to prevent them from developing. In addition, they must
recognize that environmental problems may differ in nature and magnitude in different regions; an approach that has proved successful for
controlling a problem under one set of circumstances may prove totally inadequate under another.

Environmental health professionals cannot solve these problems by themselves. They need support from legislators to pass laws, mandate regulations, and allocate funds for the development and enforcement of programs to evaluate and control various pollutants. They need support from public health educators to promote public participation in the development of programs and to ensure that regulations and requirements are fully understood by industrial organizations and other groups who are expected to comply. And they need support from program planners and economists to assure that inevitably limited funds will be spent in the most effective way.

Even more, environmental health professionals need support from the society at large. The success of any program depends on the committed action of individuals. These individuals can reduce the production of solid waste by routinely recycling newspapers, plastics, glass bottles, and aluminum cans. They can reduce energy consumption by carpooling and by installing storm windows and other weatherproofing devices. They can conserve water by using low-flow shower heads, adding a brick to the tank of a toilet to reduce the volume of water used per flush, and promptly replacing washers in leaking faucets.

There are many organizations through which people can work to bring about corrective action at the local, state, federal, and international levels. In the United States, these include the Audubon Society, the Environmental Defense Fund, Greenpeace, the League of Women Voters, the National Wildlife Federation, the Natural Resources Defense Council, the Public Interest Research Groups, the Sierra Club, and the Union of Concerned Scientists. The building of grass-roots support is often a major stimulus for actions by state legislatures and the U.S. Congress.

The General Outlook

The 1990s may well become known as the decade of the environment. Oil spills of catastrophic proportions, devastating air pollution in eastern Europe, the fouling of beaches with medical waste, the rapid destruction of rain forests, and growing awareness of the potential impacts of the "greenhouse effect" and the destruction of the ozone layer have focused public and governmental attention on the urgent need to clean up and protect the environment. These events illustrate how closely the health of humans, other animals, and plants, the survival of historical landmarks, and the beauty of the sky and countryside, depend upon the health of the global environment. These problems have been compounded by other forms of more localized environmental degradation. These range from the presence of airborne contaminants in dwellings to the problems of disposing of solid waste, especially plastic products and nonbiodegradable materials; the cleanup of toxic chemical disposal sites; widespread environmental contamination at various facilities operated by the U.S. Department of Energy; and airborne releases associated with the use of energy and the generation of electricity.

Today, highly sophisticated and sensitive instruments can measure many environmental contaminants at concentrations well below those that have been shown to cause harm to health or the environment; measurements in the parts per billion range are common. But the capability to measure much lower concentrations should not stampede either the public or policy makers into demanding "zero" pollution. This goal is neither realistic nor achievable. Rather, the goal should be an optimal level of human and environmental well-being given the host of factors that are an integral part of our daily lives.

REFERENCES

Doll, R., and R. Peto. 1981. "The Causes of Cancer: Quantitative Estimates of Avoidable Risks of Cancer in the United States Today." *Journal of the National Cancer Institute* 66, no. 6 (June), 1191–1309.

Hahn, R. W., and E. H. Males. 1990. "Can Regulatory Institutions Cope with Cross Media Pollution?" *Journal of the Air & Waste Management Association* 40, no. 1 (January), 24–31.

Surgeon General. 1989. "Executive Summary, The Surgeon General's 1989 Report on Reducing the Health Consequences of Smoking: 25 Years of Progress." *Morbidity and Mortality Weekly Report* 38, no. S-2 (24 March), 8.

Train, Russell E. 1990. "Environmental Concerns for the Year 2000." *The Bridge* 20, no. 2 (Summer), 3–10.

2

Air in the Home and Community

People have been aware for centuries of the effects of airborne pollutants on human health. Problems stemming from air pollution were noted during the Roman Empire. In the 1300s authorities in England banned silver and armor smithing because they realized that it contributed to air pollution. In 1895, Pittsburgh passed air pollution ordinances to reduce the amount of contaminants being released by steel mills. An ordinance passed in Boston in 1911 was the first to acknowledge that air pollution has regional and national as well as local effects.

As is frequently the case, it required several major, acute episodes to demonstrate conclusively to policymakers and the public that air pollution could have significant effects on health. In 1930, for example, in Belgium's Meuse River valley, high concentrations of air pollutants held close to the ground by a thermal atmospheric inversion during a period of cold, damp weather led to the deaths of 60 people. The principal sources of pollution were industrial operations, including a zinc smelter, sulfuric acid plant, and glass factories. Most of the deaths occurred among older people with a previous history of heart and lung disease. In 1948 in Donora, Pennsylvania, another river valley, about 20 people died as a result of air pollution from iron and steel plants, zinc smelting, and an acid plant. Again, cold, damp weather was accompanied by a thermal atmospheric inversion. In London in 1952, 4,000 people died as a result of domestic coal burning during similar meteorological conditions. Most of the people admitted to hospital were older or already seriously ill, affected by shortness of breath and coughing. Similar episodes occurred in 1959 and 1962, and analyses of death records have shown that there were probably others in 1873, 1880, 1882, 1891, and 1892 (Goldsmith, 1968).

Now concern is mounting over the effects of decades of environmentally blind industrial development in eastern Europe and the Soviet Union, which appears to have produced widespread threats to health and life from air pollution (French, 1991). Although specific data are lacking, reports indicate that tens of thousands of people there have developed respiratory and cardiovascular ailments as a result of various airborne contaminants; that air pollution is so severe that drivers must use their headlights in the middle of the day; and that in many industrial areas 75 percent of children have respiratory disease (Munson, 1990). In fact, outrage over environmental pollution is said to have been a catalyst in the 1990 revolution against Communist rule in Poland (French, 1991).

Today the effects of air pollution on human health and on the global environment are widely recognized. Most industrialized nations have taken steps to prevent the occurrence of acute episodes and to limit the long-term, or chronic, health effects of airborne releases. Even so, estimates suggest that up to 8 percent of Americans suffer from chronic bronchitis, emphysema, or asthma either caused or aggravated by air pollution. The accompanying costs to society are enormous: a lower quality of life for the affected individuals, shorter life spans, and less productivity and time at work.

The Body's Responses to Air Pollution

As with all other kinds of environmental insults, the human respiratory system has a variety of protective mechanisms against air pollutants. Airborne particles that are inhaled and deposited in the lungs may be removed from the upper respiratory tract by mucociliary action, or they may be engulfed and destroyed in the lower parts of the lungs by cells called macrophages. Usually the cilia sweep these, along with dirt and bacteria-laden mucus, upward to the esophagus, where they are expectorated or swallowed. Exposure to airborne gaseous irritants may cause sneezing or coughing and thus prevent their entry into the deep parts of the lungs. The body has mechanisms for detoxifying most gases taken into the lungs and absorbed. A notable exception is carbon monoxide. Where the detoxification takes place depends on how soluble the gas is in various tissues and organs, and how and with what it reacts chemically.

Despite these mechanisms, some materials will still be deposited in the body. If they remain in the lungs, they may cause constant or recurrent irritation and lead to long-term damage there. If carried by the bloodstream to other parts of the body, they can cause chronic damage to organs such as the spleen, kidneys, or liver.

Nature and Sources of Air Pollution

Air pollution has been defined as the presence in the air of substances in concentrations sufficient to interfere with health, comfort, safety, or the full use and enjoyment of property. As such, substances released into the air are considered potential pollutants not only in terms of their effects on human health but also in terms of their effects on agricultural products and on buildings, statues, and other public landmarks. In fact studies show that far lower concentrations of some air pollutants will damage agricultural products (so-called secondary standards) than concentrations considered acceptable for humans (so-called primary standards).

Air pollution can be produced by both stationary and mobile sources, both outdoors and indoors, and can lead not only to acute and chronic health problems but also to long-term global effects. For example, scientists are concerned that the discharge of carbon dioxide into the atmosphere could lead to a warming of the earth known as the "greenhouse effect" and that continued releases of chlorofluoro-carbons could destroy the stratospheric ozone layer; they already know that acidic deposition is produced by releases of nitrogen and sulfur oxides into the atmosphere. These macroscopic phenomena are discussed further in Chapter 14.

Outdoor air pollutants come in a wide range of particulates (such as soot and metallic oxides) and gases (such as carbon monoxide, nitrogen and sulfur oxides, and hydrocarbons), each with its own chemical and physical properties. Sunlight can produce a series of chemical reactions in compounds such as nitrogen oxides and hydro-carbons and convert them into secondary pollutants, such as photo-chemical oxidants. Ozone, the most abundant photochemical oxidant, is one of the most interesting atmospheric pollutants. At ground level it contributes to urban smog, and when inhaled it can exacerbate asthma and reduce the lungs' ability to remove infectious agents and toxins. Ozone also interferes with photosynthesis, causing reduced yields of agricultural crops and retarded growth in sensitive tree species. In the stratosphere, however, ozone provides an essential shield against excess ultraviolet light reaching the earth from the sun. Reductions in concentrations of stratospheric ozone can lead to increased levels of ultraviolet light and accompanying skin cancers in people, as well as damage to forests, crops, and wildlife.

Table 2.1 summarizes the relative contributions of various sources to five categories of airborne emissions in the United States in 1989: particulate matter, sulfur oxides, carbon monoxide, nitrogen oxides, and volatile organics (hydrocarbons). The principal industrial source of particulates and sulfur dioxide is the burning of fossil fuels in power (electricity-generating) plants. Automobiles are a major source of carbon monoxide, nitrogen oxides, and volatile organics, but hydrocarbons are also released by petroleum refineries, solvent manufacturers, and distributors and users of their products, such as gasoline stations and dry cleaners. Various industrial operations (including smelters, mills, refineries, and factories) also produce a wide range of particulates and vapors, including compounds containing arsenic, asbestos, beryllium, cadmium, and mercury. The relative quantities of these pollutants vary geographically. For example, emissions and airborne concentrations of carbon monoxide, nitrogen oxides, and hydrocarbons are higher in urban areas because of the greater number of motor vehicles and greater use of dry-cleaning fluids and industrial solvents; motor vehicles alone can account for 50 percent or more of urban releases of nitrogen oxides.

Control of Air Pollution

The best way to control air pollution is to prevent it in the first place, by altering the processes that produce it or by substituting nonpolluting substances for those that generate pollutants. An excellent example of this approach is the ban in the United States on the use of lead in gasoline. Some controls can be implemented on a generic basis. For example, installation of emission-control devices in automobiles is required as part of the manufacturing process. And for major industrial operations (such as power stations, solid-waste incinerators, and metallurgical plants) that have uniform characteristics, emission controls can be specified nationwide by federal regulations.

Other controls must be tailored to a wide range of characteristics, such as the size of the operation, the processes used, and the age and

Table 2.1   Sources of pollutant emissions, United States, 1989

Source	Particulate matter[a]		Sulfur oxides		Carbon monoxide		Nitrogen oxides		Volatile organics	
	10^6 tons	%	10^6 tons	%	10^6 tons	%	10^6 tons	%	10^6 tons	%
Transportation	1.5	25	1.0	5	40.0	66	7.9	40	6.4	35
Fuel combustion	1.3	22	16.8	80	7.8	13	11.1	56	0.9	5
Industrial processes	2.3	39	3.3	16	4.6	8	0.6	3	8.1	44
Solid waste	0.2	3	0.0	0	1.7	3	0.1	1	0.6	3
Miscellaneous	0.7	12	0.0	0	6.7	11	0.2	1	2.5	14
Total	5.9		21.1		60.9		19.9		18.5	

Note: Because of rounding, the totals may not represent the sum of the individual source contributions; similarly, the percentages may not add to 100.

a. Since 1987, particulate matter smaller than 10 micrometers has been reported instead of total suspended particulates to represent more closely airborne particles in the respirable range. Natural and nontraditional sources (such as agricultural tilling, mining and quarrying, and wind erosion) contribute far more airborne particulates than the sources tabulated here.

condition of the facility. Many of these are similar to the approaches used to control airborne contaminants in the workplace (Chapter 3). Approaches for controlling the releases of air pollutants from industrial and commercial operations include:

Dilute in the atmosphere: This minimal form of control uses the dilution capacity of the local atmosphere to reduce the concentrations of a pollutant to an acceptable level. In many cases it simply spreads the risk over a larger area. This approach can be applied only if the amount of pollution and the number of sources in the area are limited and if regulations permit it.

Prevent formation: This approach either eliminates the pollutant by substituting materials or methods that do not produce it, or limits the amounts of key chemical elements available for pollutant production. Examples are using substitutes for lead to improve the octane rating of gasoline, and limiting the permissible sulfur content in coal and oil burned in electric power plants.

Reduce the quantity: Examples of this approach include improving the combustion efficiency of furnaces, adding exhaust and emission controls to motor vehicles, and keeping automobiles properly tuned to minimize their emissions.

Change the process or equipment: Examples of this approach are the use of fully enclosed systems in processes that generate vapors, the use of floating covers on volatile-fluid storage tanks, and the use of electric motors instead of gasoline engines.

Apply air-cleaning technologies: Examples of this approach are the use of filters, electrostatic precipitators, scrubbers, adsorbers, or some combination of these to remove pollutants from airborne exhaust systems.

These control approaches are primarily technical. There are also many ways to reduce air pollution through changes in lifestyle. Examples include using economic incentives to promote mass transportation and carpooling; applying land-use management techniques to restrict certain areas to residential, commercial, or industrial use; and promoting the use of products that are readily recycled.

Many of the control approaches described above have been mandated by federal legislation and subsequently implemented through regulations promulgated by the U.S. Environmental Protection Agency (EPA) in cooperation with state and local environmental and

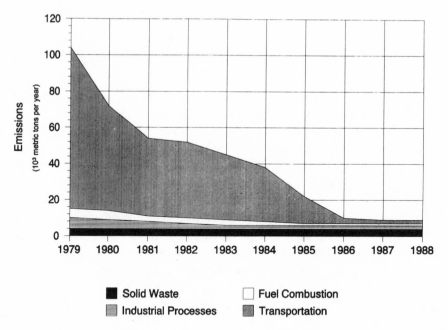

Figure 2.1   Annual airborne emissions of lead, United States, 1979–1988

regulatory agencies. These efforts have significantly reduced many sources of air pollution in the United States. For example, in 1989 automobiles manufactured since 1982 accounted for 57 percent of miles traveled, but for only 16 percent of vehicular emissions of hydrocarbons and carbon monoxide and for only 28 percent of nitrogen oxides (General Motors, 1990).

In implementing its control program, the EPA has designated National Ambient Air Quality Standards (NAAQSs) for six pollutants: particulate matter, sulfur dioxide, carbon monoxide, nitrogen oxides, volatile organic compounds, and lead. Figures 2.1, 2.2, and 2.3 show the estimated annual emissions of lead, sulfur oxides, and volatile organic compounds, by source, in the United States for the years 1979–1988. The dramatic decline in lead emissions reflects the ban on its use in gasoline.

These figures and the data in Table 2.2 reflect significant progress nationwide in reducing ambient concentrations and releases of all six pollutants except for volatile organic compounds which lead to the

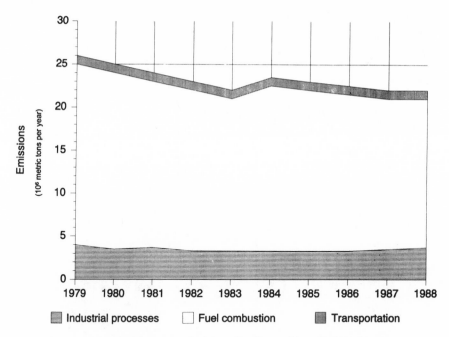

Figure 2.2. Annual airborne emissions of sulfur oxides, United States, 1979–1988

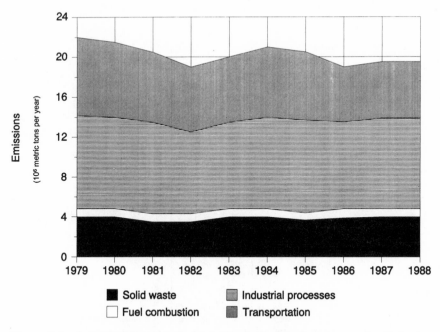

Figure 2.3 Annual airborne emissions of volatile organic compounds, United States, 1979–1988

Table 2.2 Sources, annual emissions, removal mechanisms, and trends in concentrations of key atmospheric pollutants, United States

| Pollutant | Major source | | Estimated annual emission, 1988 (10^6 tons/year) | | Removal mechanism | Estimated time in atmosphere | % change, 1979–1988 | |
	Natural	Man-made	Natural	Man-made			Source emission	Airborne concentration
Particulate matter	Volcanoes, wind erosion, pollens, forest fires	Industrial processes, combustion, transportation	25–300	7.5	Larger particles settle to earth; smaller particles brought down with precipitation	Minutes to a few days	−22	−20 (geometric mean for 175 sites)
Sulfur dioxide	Volcanoes, reactions of biogenic sulfur emissions	Fossil fuel combustion	2	21	Oxidation of sulfate by photochemical reactions and incorporation into precipitation	1–4 days	−17	−30 (arithmetic mean for 374 sites)

Carbon monoxide	Transportation, general combustion	210	Forest fires, photochemical reactions	65	Photochemical reactions with CH_4 and OH	1–3 months	−25	−28 (second-highest 8-hour average for 248 sites)
Nitrogen oxides	Combustion	18[a]	Lightning, biogenic processes in soil	20	Oxidation to nitrate and incorporation into precipitation	2–5 days	−8	−7 (annual mean for NO_2 at 116 sites)
Volatile organic compounds	Combustion, transportation	0.2–1	Biogenic processes in soil and vegetation	18	Photochemical reactions with NO and ozone	Hours to a few days	−17	+2 (second-highest daily 1-hour maximum for ozone at 388 sites)
Lead	Transportation, fuel combustion, lead smelting and refining, storage-battery manufacturing	(−)	Wind-blown soil	0.007	Larger particles settle to earth; smaller particles brought down with precipitation	Minutes to a few days	−93	−89 (maximum quarterly average at 139 sites)

a. As NO_2.

production of ozone. Moreover, these reductions occurred during a time of continued industrial and population growth. But the results vary by city and by region. According to EPA estimates, for example, in 1988 121 million people in the United States still resided in counties that did not meet even one NAAQS. Ground-level ozone appears to be the most pervasive problem: the 112 million people living in counties that exceeded the ozone standard in 1988 outnumbered the total population in all the areas in which the standards for the other five pollutants were exceeded (EPA, 1990).

The Clean Air Act Amendments of 1990 have strengthened air pollution control measures in the United States. For one thing, operating permits are now required for stationary sources of air pollution (Lee, 1991). This change follows policies that have proved successful in the control of water pollution sources. Another concept established by the law is a system of tradable emissions credits: now the operator of an industrial facility who reduces emissions below the standard or ahead of the timetable set by the law earns emission credits that can be applied to future emissions or sold to an operator of another facility. Specific goals of the new amendments include still lower emission limits for cars and light trucks; additional pollution controls for oil refineries, chemical plants, gasoline stations, and dry cleaners; new controls for coal-burning electric power plants to reduce acidic deposition; and phased-out production of chemicals that contribute to depletion of the stratospheric ozone layer. The Clean Air Amendments of 1990 mandate a 50 percent reduction by the year 2000 in the pollutants, most notably sulfur dioxide, that can lead to the production of acid rain. All the other mandated reductions also have timetables for compliance.

Achieving these goals will require the use of reformulated gasoline mixtures or other sources of power, such as electricity, in motor vehicles; and, in power plants, the use of other fuels or coal with a lower sulfur content, the installation of emission controls such as scrubbers, or the application of innovative technologies such as fluidized bed plants and integrated gasification combined-cycle plants (Abelson, 1990). Other possible approaches include expanded uses of solar and nuclear power. All such strategies involve trade-offs. Efforts to reduce one type of pollutant may lead to other types of environmental and public health problems. For example, using methanol as a fuel for cars would significantly reduce hydrocarbon emissions but increase formaldehyde emissions, and using methanol as a fuel may be less cost effective than other approaches in reducing hydrocarbons (Walls and Krupnick, 1990). Similarly, the use of electric-powered automobiles would reduce airborne emissions in metropolitan areas but could lead to increased pollution from electricity-generating stations. And installing scrubbers to remove sulfur from power plants will produce large volumes of solid waste.

Indoor Air Pollution

Having made a start in reducing the concentrations of airborne pollutants in the ambient environment, environmental health professionals are directing more and more attention to the assessment and control of airborne contaminants in residential and office buildings. There are two major reasons for this broadened emphasis. First, people living in cities spend, on the average, 90 percent or more of their time indoors. Second, there is a host of potentially significant sources of indoor air pollution. In many cities, indoor concentrations of nitrogen oxides, carbon monoxide, airborne particulates, and other volatile organic compounds exceed measured outdoor pollutant concentrations. Even if indoor concentrations proved to be low, the longer duration of indoor exposures could render them significant in the total exposure of the general population.

Sources

Although indoor exposures have received attention only in the last few decades, soot found on ceilings of prehistoric caves provides evidence of millenia of such exposures. Relatively high concentrations of airborne pollutants are common where people cook over open fires fueled by charcoal, wood, coal, kerosene, or oil. In technologically advanced nations the use of synthetic materials in construction, the design of buildings to be energy efficient, and the increased use of wood- and coal-burning stoves and kerosene heaters (all of which emit toxic and carcinogenic particles and gases) have increased the quantity and complexity of airborne exposures despite code-specified ventilation requirements. Mobile homes and prefabricated housing units contribute significantly to these problems. Mobile homes currently account for about 20 percent of the new housing stock, and this trend is expected to accelerate as restrictions in zoning laws are phased out in many localities. Mobile homes and prefabricated housing have smaller volumes and lower air-exchange rates, are constructed of more materials containing volatile organic resins, and are more likely to use propane as a cooking fuel than conventionally built dwellings (Spengler and Sexton, 1983).

There are six major sources of indoor air pollution.

Combustion By-Products

Combustion of fuels can produce and release carbon monoxide, carbon dioxide, sulfur dioxide, formaldehyde, hydrocarbons, nitrogen oxides, and a variety of airborne particles. Depending on the source and type of fuel and the air-exchange rate, long-term indoor average nitrogen dioxide concentrations can exceed the National Ambient Air Quality Standards. For example, peak hourly nitrogen dioxide concentrations from conventional gas cooking may range from two to seven times the NAAQS. Airborne nitrogen dioxide and carbon monoxide have been found in homes and schools using unvented kerosene and gas heaters, and in skating arenas where gasoline powered ice-cleaning equipment is used (Spengler and Sexton, 1983).

Such contaminants can have both chronic and acute effects. Elevated exposures to nitrogen dioxide are associated with chronic toxicological effects, including pulmonary edema, bronchoconstriction, and increased infection rates. Similar exposure to carbon monoxide from faulty furnaces and attached garages can result in asphyxiation.

Microorganisms and Allergens

Pets, detergents, humidifiers, air-cooling towers, and insects that live in dust and ventilation ducts can release pollens, molds, mites, chemical additives, animal dander, fungi, algae, and insect parts. Air-cooling equipment, cool-mist vaporizers, humidifiers, nebulizers, flush toilets, ice machines, and carpeting can incubate and distribute airborne bacteria indoors. Related bacterial infections include legionnaire's disease and humidifier fever. Ultrasonic humidifiers using tap water can dispense minerals into the air in the form of aerosolized droplets (Highsmith, Rodes, and Hardy, 1988). These droplets evaporate into particles small enough to enter the lungs, causing respiratory irritation and associated health problems. Tightly sealed buildings in humid climates enhance the growth of molds and fungi. Reduced ventilation rates and untreated recirculated air also tend to increase the airborne concentrations of microorganisms in buildings (Spengler and Sexton, 1983).

Formaldehyde and Other Organic Compounds

Formaldehyde is a common ingredient in many building materials (such as plywood and particle board), in furnishings (such as draperies and carpets), and in some types of foam insulation. Excess formaldehyde in such products can continue to be released over several years. Other sources of formaldehyde include unvented gas combustion units and tobacco smoke. Low concentrations can cause eye discomfort; higher concentrations can cause lower respiratory irritation and pulmonary edema and may also affect the central nervous system, producing subtle changes in short-term memory, increased anxiety, and slight changes in the ability to adapt to darkness (Spengler and Sexton, 1983).

Other sources of organic contaminants in indoor environments include the combustion of wood, kerosene, and tobacco products, which yield polycyclic aromatic hydrocarbons; and personal-care products, cleaning materials, paints, lacquers, and varnishes, which generate chlorinated compounds, acetone, ammonia, toluene, and benzene (Spengler and Sexton, 1983).

Asbestos Fibers

Until 1980 asbestos was used in many building materials, including ceiling and floor tiles, pipe insulation, spackling compounds, concrete, and acoustical and thermal insulation. Workers exposed to asbestos have shown increases in lung cancer, pleural and peritoneal mesotheliomas, and gastrointestinal tract cancers (Mossman et al., 1990). Several studies have also shown increased mesothelioma rates among people living near asbestos-production facilities and shipyards, and among family members of asbestos-exposed workers (Kilburn, 1990). People living or working in buildings containing asbestos, however, need to be concerned only if the asbestos is friable (shedding). In most cases, exposures are minimal. Throughout the 1980s EPA programs promoted the removal of asbestos from buildings. Experience has shown, however, that it may be safer to leave the material in place, especially if it is well contained (Mossman et al., 1990).

Tobacco Smoke

More than 2,000 compounds have been identified in cigarette smoke. Many of these are known carcinogens and irritants. Specific airborne contaminants present in cigarette smoke include respirable particles, nicotine, polycyclic aromatic hydrocarbons, carbon monoxide, acrolein, and nitrogen dioxide. Concentrations in dwellings and in public places vary widely, depending on air filtration rates, the frequency and amount of smoking, the number and use of air-cleaning devices, and the kind of ventilation system. Airborne particle concentrations in a home with several heavy smokers can exceed ambient air quality standards (Spengler and Sexton, 1983). Epidemiological studies reveal a direct correlation between the extent of maternal smoking and various reported illnesses in children (Ferris et al., 1986). Similarly, Berkey et al. (1984) reported significantly lower heights and weights in 6-to-11-year-olds whose mothers smoked.

Radon and Its Airborne Decay Products

Recent studies by the EPA and the National Council on Radiation Protection and Measurements (NCRP) have found that elevated concentrations of the naturally occurring radioactive gas radon (Rn-222) are present in many houses in the United States and are a significant source of radiation exposure. According to one estimate, radon and its airborne decay products account for 55 percent of the current radiation dose to the U.S. population (NCRP, 1987). As many as 5–10 percent of houses in the United States may have radon concentrations higher than the level at which remedial action is recommended (Figure 2.4). On the basis of epidemiological studies of uranium miners who developed lung cancer as a result of occupational exposures to airborne radon decay products, it is estimated that the presence of this contaminant in U.S. houses causes 5,000–20,000 deaths from lung cancer annually (AMA, 1987).

Table 2.3 summarizes indoor airborne contaminants, their major sources, and their concentrations relative to the ambient environment.

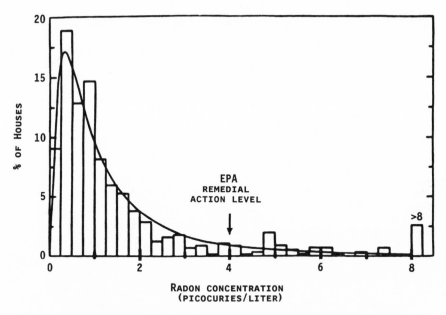

Figure 2.4   Frequency distribution of radon-222 concentrations in 552 U.S. houses

Control Measures

Control measures are available for most indoor airborne contaminants. However, effective control depends on an understanding of several factors. First, the characteristics of the contaminant (such as concentration, reactivity, physical state, and particle size) must be assessed. All such characteristics affect its removal. Second, the nature of the emissions must be ascertained. For example, are they continuous or intermittent, from single or multiple sources, and primarily inside or outside? Third, the quantitative relationship between the exposure and the resulting health effects must be considered. Are individuals to be protected primarily from long-term chronic exposures to low concentrations, or from periodic short-term exposures at peak concentrations? Finally, the nature of the facility may be important: some controls are more readily applied in residential buildings, others in commercial or office buildings. Also important are the age and condition of the building.

Table 2.3 Indoor air pollutants, sources, and indoor/outdoor concentration
ratios

Pollutant	Major source	Indoor/outdoor concentration ratio
Origin predominantly outdoors		
Sulfur oxides (gases, particles)	Fuel combustion, smelters	< 1
Ozone	Photochemical reactions	≪ 1
Pollens	Trees, grass, weeds, plants	< 1
Lead, manganese	Automobiles	< 1
Calcium, chlorine, silicon, cadmium	Suspension of soils, industrial emissions	< 1
Organic substances	Petrochemical solvents, natural sources, vaporization of unburned fuels	< 1
Origin indoors or outdoors		
Nitric oxide, nitrogen dioxide	Fuel burning	≫ 1
Carbon monoxide	Fuel burning	≫ 1
Carbon dioxide	Metabolic activity, combustion	≫ 1
Particles	Resuspension, condensation of vapors, combustion products	> 1
Water vapor	Biological activity, combustion evaporation	> 1
Organic substances	Volatilization, combustion, paint, metabolic action, pesticides	≫ 1
Spores	Fungi, molds	> 1

Table 2.3   (continued)

Pollutant	Major source	Indoor/outdoor concentration ratio
Origin predominantly indoors		
Radon	Underlying soil, water supply, building construction matrials (concrete, stone)	≫ 1
Formaldehyde	Particle board, insulation, furnishings, tobacco smoke	> 1
Asbestos, mineral, and synthetic fibers	Fire retardant materials, insulation	1
Organic substances	Adhesives, solvents, cooking, cosmetics	> 1
Ammonia	Metabolic activity, cleaning products	> 1
Polycyclic hydrocarbons, arsenic, nicotine, acrolein, etc.	Tobacco smoke	≫ 1
Mercury	Fungicides, paints, spills in dental-care facilities or labs, thermometer breakage	> 1
Aerosols	Consumer products	≫ 1
Microorganisms	People, animals, plants	> 1
Allergens	House dust, animal dander, insect parts	≫ 1

Control measures generally include a combined strategy of ventilation, source removal or substitution, source modification, air purification, and behavioral changes. Table 2.4 summarizes control methods that can be used for the more important indoor air contaminants.

Experience with radon illustrates how a better understanding of the sources and behavior of a contaminant can lead to the development of simple, inexpensive control measures. Radon, an inert gas that does not readily interact with the body, is usually released into buildings from the underlying soil. However, the solid radioactive decay products of radon, not the gas itself, are the major contributors of the dose to the lungs. When inhaled, the gas is simply exhaled, but the solid decay products may be retained in the lungs.

For dwellings in which radon concentrations are ten or more times the remedial action level (Figure 2.4), control may require building modifications such as sealing cracks in the basement floor and walls or installing a subslab exhaust system beneath the basement floor. For dwellings in which concentrations are lower, much simpler control measures are available.

The decay products of radon are solid and electrically charged. If a fan is used to circulate the air in a room so that they are brought into contact with the walls or floor, they will stick, or "plate out," and be removed from the air. Since the decay products cause health problems only if inhaled, and since air circulation generally removes at least 50 percent of the airborne decay products, this simple approach will provide effective control in dwellings with concentrations up to twice the remedial action level. If a negative- or positive-ion generator is combined with a fan, the resulting space charge will increase the deposition of airborne decay products on the walls and reduce concentrations by 80 to 90 percent. Figure 2.5 summarizes the results of laboratory evaluations of a wide range of air-cleaning approaches to the removal of airborne radon decay products.

As Figure 2.5 shows, particle-removing devices such as high-efficiency filters and electrostatic precipitators reduce the concentrations of airborne radon decay products but not the accompanying dose to the lungs. Upon being formed, the electrically charged decay products will rapidly attach themselves to any airborne dust particles in a room. A particle-removing device will keep the dust concentration low, but it will have no effect on the radon gas, which will continue to produce additional decay products. These products, in turn, will have far fewer dust particles to which to attach. Since, atom for atom, an unattached radon decay product produces 3–40 times the dose to the lungs as an identical atom that has attached itself to a dust particle (NCRP, 1984), the net result may well be no reduction, and perhaps even an increase, in the dose to the lungs. Use of electrostatic precipitators and high-efficiency filters may increase the dose by as much as 150 percent (Figure 2.5). Negative-ion generators appear to produce

Table 2.4   Control measures for indoor air pollutants

Control measure	Pollutants	Example
Ventilation: dilution of indoor air with fresh outdoor air or recirculated filtered air, using mechanical or natural methods	Radon and radon progeny, combustion by-products, tobacco smoke, biological agents (particles)	Exhaust canopy to vent gas-stove emissions; air-to-air heat exchangers for ventilation with energy conservation
Source removal or substitution: removal of indoor emission sources or substitution of less hazardous materials	Organic substances, asbestiform minerals, tobacco smoke	Restrictions on smoking in public places; removal of asbestos
Source modification: reduction of emission rates through changes in design or processes; containment of emissions by barriers or sealants	Radon and radon progeny, organic substances, asbestiform minerals, combustion by-products	Plastic barriers to reduce radon levels; containment of asbestos; catalytic oxidation of CO to CO_2 in unvented kerosene burners
Air cleaning: purification of indoor air by gas adsorbers, air filters, ion generators, and electrostatic precipitators	Particulate matter, combustion by-products, biological agents (particles), airborne radon decay products	Residential air cleaners to control tobacco smoke or wood smoke; formaldehyde-sorbent filters; fan-ion generators to remove airborne radon decay products
Behavioral adjustment: reduction in human exposure through modification of behavior patterns; facilitated by consumer education, product labeling, building design, warning devices, and legal liability	Organic substances, combustion by-products, tobacco smoke	Smoke-free zones; architectural design of interior space; certification of formaldehyde and radon concentrations for home purchases

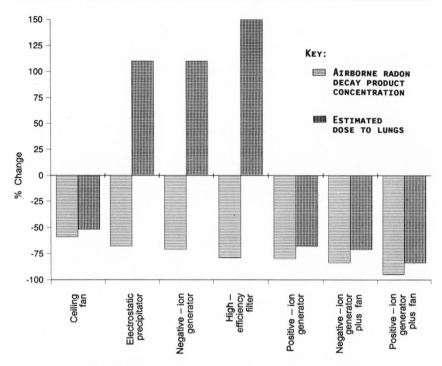

Figure 2.5 Effectiveness of various air-cleaning methods in reducing concentrations of airborne radon decay products and estimated doses to the lungs

a similar result (Maher, Rudnick, and Moeller, 1987). In light of this paradox, the EPA does not recommend the use of filtration systems to control airborne radon decay products in houses. Fortunately, either a fan alone or a fan in combination with a negative- or positive-ion generator reduces both the concentration of decay products and the dose to the lungs, and at a low cost.

The General Outlook

Despite significant progress in reducing the concentrations of some air contaminants in the ambient environment, much work remains to be done, especially in connection with long-term problems such as acidic deposition, global warming, and depletion of the ozone layer. But even if the outdoor air were pollution free, indoor air pollutants would remain causes for concern. Legislation to control indoor releases is unlikely to be enforceable, both because of the sheer number of housing units and because of the long-established principle of the sanctity of private dwellings. Only intensive public education is likely to bring reductions in existing dwellings. The best long-term approach will be to incorporate control measures in new building design, construction, and related appliances.

REFERENCES

Abelson, Philip H. 1990. "New Technology for Cleaner Air." Editorial, *Science* 248, no. 4957 (18 May), 793.

AMA, Council on Scientific Affairs. 1987. "Radon in Homes." *Journal of the American Medical Association* 258, no. 5 (7 August), 668–672.

Berkey, C. S., J. H. Ware, F. E. Speizer, and B. G. Ferris, Jr. 1984. "Passive Smoking and Height Growth of Preadolescent Children." *International Journal of Epidemiology* 13, no. 4, 454–458.

EPA. 1990. *National Air Quality and Emissions Trends Report, 1988.* Report EPA-450/4-90-002. Washington, D.C.

Ferris, B. G., Jr., J. H. Ware, J. D. Spengler, D. W. Dockery, and F. E. Speizer. 1986. "The Harvard Six-Cities Study." In *Aerosols: Research, Risk Assessment and Control Strategies.* Proceedings of the Second U.S.-Dutch International Symposium, Williamsburg, Va., 19–25 May 1985. Chelsea, Mich.: Lewis Publishers.

French, Hilary F. 1991. "Eastern Europe's Clean Break With the Past." *World-Watch* 4, no. 2 (March–April), 21–27.

General Motors Corporation. 1990. "GM and the Global Environment: An Update." In *General Motors Public Interest Report, 1990.* Detroit.

Goldsmith, J. R. 1968. "Effects of Air Pollution on Human Health." In *Air Pollution,* vol. 1: *Air Pollution and Its Effects,* ed. Arthur C. Stern. 2d ed. New York: Academic Press.

Highsmith, V. R., C. E. Rodes, and R. J. Hardy. 1988. "Indoor Particle Concentrations Associated with Use of Tap Water in Portable Humidifiers." *Environmental Science & Technology* 22, no. 9 (September), 1109.

Kilburn, Kaye H. 1990. "A Case for Ending Use of Asbestos." *Forum for Applied Research and Public Policy* 5, no. 4 (Winter), 87–89.

Lee, Bryan. 1991. "Highlights of the Clean Air Act Amendments of 1990." *Journal of the Air & Waste Management Association* 41, no. 1 (January), 16–19.

Maher, E. F., S. N. Rudnick, and D. W. Moeller. 1987. "Effective Removal of Airborne ^{222}Rn Decay Products inside Buildings." *Health Physics* 53, no. 4 (October), 351–356.

Mossman, B. T., J. Bignon, M. Corn, A. Seaton, and J. B. L. Gee. 1990. "Asbestos: Scientific Developments and Implications for Public Policy." *Science* 247, no. 4940 (19 January), 294–301.

Munson, Halsey. 1990. "Pollution in the Soviet Union." *ECON: Environmental Contractor* 5, no. 8 (August), 24–29.

NCRP. 1984. *Evaluation of Occupational and Environmental Exposures to Radon and Radon Daughters in the United States.* Report no. 78. Bethesda, Md.

—— 1987. *Ionizing Radiation Exposure of the Population of the United States.* Report no. 93. Bethesda, Md.

Spengler, J. D., and K. Sexton. 1983. "Indoor Air Pollution: A Public Health Perspective." *Science* 221, no. 4605 (1 July), 9–17.

Walls, Margaret A., and Alan J. Krupnick. 1990. "Cost-Effectiveness of Methanol Vehicles." *Resources,* no. 100 (Summer), 1–5.

3

The Workplace

As early as the fourth century B.C., Hippocrates apparently observed adverse effects on miners and metallurgists from exposures to lead. In 1473 Ulrich Ellenbog recognized that the fumes of some metals were dangerous and suggested preventive measures. In 1556 Georg Bauer (known as Georgius Agricola), a physician and mineralogist, attributed lung disease among miners in the Carpathian Mountains to the inhalation of certain kinds of mineral dusts, observing that so many miners succumbed to the disease that some women there married as many as seven times (Patty, 1978). In 1700 Bernadino Ramazzini published the first complete treatise on occupational diseases, *De Morbis Artificum Diatriba*. In the mid-1880s Karl Bernhard Lehmann, whose work continues to serve as a guide on the effects of exposures to airborne contaminants, conducted experiments on the toxic effects of gases and vapors on animals (Patty, 1978). During the same period the first occupational cancer, scrotal cancer in chimney sweeps, was observed in England.

In the United States occupational health problems received little attention until the twentieth century. The U.S. Bureau of Labor was created in 1885, but even when it became the Department of Labor in 1913 its stated goals included no mention of workers' health beyond "promoting their material, social, intellectual, and moral prosperity." And Alice Hamilton's classic work, *Exploring the Dangerous Trades,* now perhaps the most widely quoted book on the field in the world, was not published until 1943.

Protective Legislation

Protective legislation came piecemeal and slowly (Table 3.1). In 1908 the federal government provided limited compensation to civil service

Table 3.1 Significant federal legislation pertaining to occupational
health and safety

Year	Act	Content
1908	Federal Workers' Compensation Act	Granted limited compensation benefits to certain U.S. civil service workers for injuries sustained during employment
1936	Walsh-Healey Public Contracts Act	Established occupational health and safety standards for employees of federal contractors
1969	Federal Coal Mine Health and Safety Act	Created forerunner of Mine Safety and Health Administration; required development and enforcement of regulations for protection of mine workers
1970	Occupational Safety and Health Act	Authorized the federal government to develop and set mandatory occupational safety and health standards; established the National Institute for Occupational Safety and Health to conduct research for setting standards
1976	Toxic Substances Control Act	Required data from industry on production, use, and health and environmental effects of chemicals; led to development of "right-to-know" laws, which provide employees with information on the nature of potential occupational exposures

employees injured on the job. In 1911 New Jersey became the first
state to enact a workers' compensation law, but although many other
states rapidly followed suit, it was not until 1948 that all the states
required such compensation (Patty, 1978).

Workers' compensation laws, which were passed in France, Germany, and the United Kingdom in the nineteenth century, were one of the earliest forms of social insurance on a prepaid basis, with no direct monetary contribution from workers. By removing the determination of compensation for occupational injuries from the courts, these laws revolutionized the approach to the control of workplace hazards and did more than any other measure to reduce occupational injuries in the United States. Eventually some states expanded their laws to include a full range of occupational diseases and required that compensation for occupational injuries be paid on a no-fault basis, that settlements be reached promptly through administrative tribunals, and that payments be made in accordance with a system of scheduled benefits.

The Walsh-Healey Public Contracts Act of 1936 established safety and health standards in industries conducting work under contract to the federal government. This forerunner of modern occupational health regulations stimulated research on occupational disease and the development of occupational health programs by state and local agencies, insurance companies, foundations, management, and unions (Cralley and Konn, 1973). The first significant federal legislation for workers outside government projects did not come until 1969, with the Federal Coal Mine Health and Safety Act. This legislation was followed by the landmark Occupational Safety and Health Act of 1970, whose announced principal purpose was to "assure so far as possible every working man and woman in the Nation healthful working conditions and to preserve human resources." It established the Occupational Safety and Health Administration (OSHA) in the Department of Labor to encourage reduction of workplace hazards, provide for occupational and health research, establish separate but dependent responsibilities and rights for employers and employees, maintain a reporting and recordkeeping system to monitor job injuries, establish training programs, develop mandatory safety and health standards, and provide for development and approval of state occupational safety and health programs.

The Occupational Safety and Health Act also created the National Institute for Occupational Safety and Health (NIOSH) in the U.S. Department of Health and Human Services. NIOSH was made responsible for conducting research on which new occupational health standards could be based and for implementing education and training programs to provide an adequate supply of people to implement and enforce the 1970 act. As a result, epidemiologic and laboratory research into the causes of occupational diseases and injuries and ways to prevent them was expanded, and regional centers were established at several leading universities to provide training for occupational health and safety professionals. Unfortunately, funding for these programs declined after a promising start.

In recognition of the fact that proper training and education of workers, employers, and upper-level management can promote effective control of occupational health hazards, "right-to-know" provisions in amendments to the 1976 Toxic Substances Control Act required employers to furnish workers with information about the health hazards of their occupational environment.

Identifying Occupational Health Problems

Today well over 100 million men and women are gainfully employed in the United States, and increasing numbers of people, particularly women, are entering the work force. All these workers are exposed to some degree to occupational hazards, and all risk job-related adverse health effects. Compounding these problems is the fact that more than 25 percent of Americans are employed in businesses that have fewer than 20 employees, and more than 50 percent in companies with fewer than 100 employees. These smaller companies often lack the knowledge to identify occupational health hazards and the funds to finance associated control programs; moreover, many are exempt from state and federal occupational health and safety regulations.

The effects of occupational exposures range from lung diseases, cancer, hearing loss, and dermatitis to more subtle psychological effects, many of which are only now beginning to be recognized (Table 3.2). Workplace exposures include airborne contaminants, ionizing radiation, ultraviolet and visible light, electric and magnetic fields, infrared radiation, microwaves, heat, cold, noise, extremes of barometric pressure, and stress-related effects. Each of these may also interact with other chemical, physical, or biological agents. For example, cardiovascular diseases may be related to a combination of physical, chemical, and psychological job stresses. The workplace can also be a source of a wide range of infectious diseases. Hospital workers, especially, must be concerned with protection against hepatitis B, tuberculosis, influenza, and other viral infections, including acquired immune deficiency syndrome (AIDS).

Table 3.2   The 10 leading work-related diseases and injuries,
United States, 1990

Type of disorder or injury	Examples
Occupational lung diseases	Asbestosis, byssinosis, silicosis, coal workers' pneumoconiosis, lung cancer, occupational asthma
Musculoskeletal injuries	Disorders of the back, trunk, upper extremity, neck, lower extremity; traumatically induced Raynaud's phenomenon
Occupational cancers (other than lung)	Leukemia, mesothelioma, cancers of the bladder, nose, and liver
Severe occupational injuries	Amputations, fractures, eye loss, lacerations, traumatic deaths
Cardiovascular diseases	Hypertension, coronary artery disease, acute myocardial infarction
Reproductive disorders	Infertility, spontaneous abortion, teratogenesis
Neurotoxic disorders	Peripheral neuropathy, toxic encephalitis, psychoses, extreme personality changes
Noise-induced loss of hearing	
Dermatologic conditions	Dermatoses, burns, chemical burns, contusions
Psychological disorders	Neuroses, personality disorders, alcoholism, drug dependency

Toxic chemicals, widely used in industry, play a major role in occupationally related diseases. The two major portals of entry for such agents are the skin and the respiratory tract. Once inside the body, toxic agents can affect other organs, such as the liver and kidneys.

The National Safety Council (1990) estimates that about 100,000 new cases of job-related illnesses occur annually in the United States. Industrial accidents account for another 1.7 million disabling injuries and some 10,000–12,000 deaths. The costs associated with accidental deaths and injuries—loss of wages, medical expenses, insurance administrative costs, fire losses, and other indirect expenses—are esti-

mated to approach $50 billion per year. Insurance data indicate that
people in certain higher-risk occupations, such as agriculture, construction, mining, and quarrying, have three to four times the average
death rate for all industries (National Safety Council, 1990).

Large though these numbers are, the true magnitude of the health
and economic impacts of occupational disease and injury remains un-
known, for several reasons. First, the recording of data on workers'
illnesses and deaths is often incomplete or erroneous. Physicians frequently fail to relate observed diseases to occupational exposures.
This is particularly true for neurologically based illnesses (Weiss,
1990) and for chronic degenerative diseases such as atherosclerosis
and chronic obstructive respiratory ailments. In other cases, the cause
of death even if diagnosed is nòt coded into the death certificate. Even
when the required information is available, it may not be used to
promote worker protection. Second, because the health effects of
chronic exposures to various toxic agents in the workplace are delayed, and because many workers change jobs frequently, by the time
a disease manifests itself it may be very difficult to relate it to a
specific exposure or combination of exposures. Third, even if an association between a specific disease and a given toxic agent is known,
it is often difficult to quantify the concentration of the toxic agent to
which the worker was exposed and to measure the intake of toxic
agents and the accompanying dose.

Economic considerations also tend to delay or reduce attempts to
solve occupational health problems. In large corporations, the direc-
tors and officers acting on behalf of stockholders may insist on operating industrial facilities with a primary view to profits rather than
to occupational health. For example, they may insist that a refinery
be kept in operation, with minimum time for shutdowns for maintenance or overhaul, at the expense of worker health and safety. Moreover, workers themselves frequently object to controls designed to
enhance health and safety when such measures slow production or
interfere with comfort. This is especially true in times of economic
recession, when many people fear losing their jobs. In addition, there
is a chronic shortage of people qualified to investigate and control
exposures in industry. Federal funding for training professional occupational health personnel has been declining, and the overall shortage
of funds for regulatory organizations has reduced the number and
frequency of OSHA inspections in workplaces.

Another problem is that the patterns of occupational disease are constantly changing, requiring ever-more-refined methods to uncover the subtle injuries and disabilities resulting from low-level on-the-job psychological stress and other nonphysical or chemical hazards. Conducting more dose-response studies entails not only training more professionals in the necessary disciplines but also developing better recordkeeping and health data systems to facilitate epidemiological studies. Also needed are more reliable animal models for predicting human effects, earlier indicators of diseases as they develop, and improved environmental and biological monitoring procedures.

Unless these problems are solved, it will continue to be difficult to identify occupational hazards, determine their magnitude, and judge the adequacy of control measures. The success of these efforts has implications far beyond the occupational environment: because concentrated exposures to hazardous agents frequently occur first in the workplace, and the associated health effects are initially identified and observed among workers, the monitoring of occupational exposures can, and often does, provide the first warning of the presence of potential hazards in the general environment. Clearly, occupational diseases and injuries have consequences not only for workers but also for their families and their communities.

Obviously, the ideal way to control exposure to toxic chemicals is to assess their toxicological risk before they are introduced into the workplace (Burgess, 1981). Despite advances in "predictive" toxicology, much work needs to be done to develop practical and reliable screening systems to identify chemicals that have potential for harming human health.

Occupational Exposure Standards

The late 1930s brought the first organizations of occupational health professionals and, with them, the first occupational health and safety standards. The American Conference of Governmental Industrial Hygienists (ACGIH), established in 1938, has played a major role in developing limits for exposures in the workplace. Early on, it established "threshold limit values" (TLVs) providing guidance on permissible concentrations of airborne contaminants (Table 3.3). TLVs now exist for more than 600 chemical substances. The American Industrial Hygiene Association (established in 1939), OSHA, and NIOSH have

Table 3.3   Threshold limit values for selected chemical substances in air

Substance	Typical industrial uses or sources	Time-weighted average[a]		Short-term exposure limit[b]	
		ppm[c]	mg/m^3	ppm[c]	mg/m^3
Ammonia	Coke ovens	25	17	35	24
Benzene	Gasoline refining, organic chemical synthesizing	10	32	—	—
Carbon monoxide	Blast furnaces, coal mines	50	57	400	458
Chlorine	Fabric bleaching, water purification	0.5	1.5	1	2.9
Formaldehyde	Embalming, pathology	1	1.2	2	2.5
Lead (inorganic dusts and fumes)	Battery manufacturing	—	0.15	—	—
Toluene	Lacquer manufacturing, petroleum refining	100	377	150	565
Trichloroethylene	Metal degreasing	50	269	200	1070
Vinyl acetate	Artificial leather manufacturing	10	35	20	70

a. For normal 8-hour day, 40-hour workweek.
b. Not to exceed 15 minutes more than four times per day.
c. Parts per million.

essentially followed the ACGIH in developing their workplace exposure limits. Recently the ACGIH has provided biological exposure indexes for about two dozen chemicals. Indexes for selected chemicals are shown in Table 3.4.

By establishing both TLVs and exposure indexes, the ACGIH offers a two-step approach to the assessment of the importance of chemicals in the workplace: first, monitoring of the air being breathed; second, monitoring of the chemicals themselves or their metabolites in biological specimens (such as urine, blood, and exhaled air) collected from workers at specified intervals. The first step provides data

Table 3.4 Biological exposure indexes for selected airborne chemicals

Chemical	Sampling time	Biological exposure index
Benzene		
Total phenol in urine	End of shift	50 mg/liter
Benzene in exhaled air	Before next shift	
Mixed-exhaled[a]		0.08 ppm
End-exhaled[b]		0.12 ppm
Carbon monoxide		
Carboxyhemoglobin in blood	End of shift	< 8% of hemoglobin
CO in end-exhaled air[b]	End of shift	< 40 ppm
Lead		
Lead in blood	Not critical	50 μg/100 ml
Lead in urine	Not critical	150 μg/g creatinine
Zinc protoporphyrin in blood	After 1 month exposure	250 μg/100 ml erythrocytes or 100 μg/100 ml blood
Toluene		
Hippuric acid in urine	End of shift	2.5 g/g creatinine
	Last 4 hours of shift	3 mg/min
Toluene in venous blood	End of shift	1 mg/liter
Toluene in end-exhaled air[b]	During shift	20 ppm
Trichloroethylene		
Trichloroacetic acid in urine	End of workweek	100 mg/liter
Trichloroacetic acid and trichloroethanol in urine	End of shift at end of workweek	300 mg/liter 320 mg/g creatinine
Free tricholoethanol in blood	End of shift at end of workweek	4 mg/liter
Trichloroethylene in end-exhaled air[b]	Prior to last shift of workweek	0.5 ppm

Note: ppm = parts per million.
a. Combination or mixture of air from upper and lower respiratory system.
b. Usually represents alveolar air from lower respiratory system.

Table 3.5   Threshold limit values for noise in the workplace

Typical industrial source	Exposure time (hours per day)	Sound level (decibels)
Textile plants, forge shops, machine shops,	1/8	115[a]
jackhammer operators	1/4	110
	1/2	105
	1	100
	2	95
	4	90
	8	85
	16	80

a. No exposure should be permitted to continuous or intermittent sound levels in excess of 115 decibels.

on exposures to workers; the second step provides data on the resulting doses. Although there is generally a close correlation between these two sets of measurements, the resulting data are not synonymous. Exposures are indicators of conditions in the working environment; doses are indicators of how much of a given contaminant has been taken into the body. Since exposures can be measured without intruding on the privacy of the worker, exposures are generally used as a surrogate for doses.

The ACGIH has also developed recommendations for limiting concentrations of explosive gases and for assessing the safety of confined spaces before standby personnel enter them to rescue a worker who has succumbed to a hazardous environment. And it has established TLVs for physical agents, including heat and cold, noise (Table 3.5), vibration, lasers, radiofrequency/microwave radiation, magnetic fields, and ultraviolet and ionizing radiation (ACGIH, 1990).

TLVs are based on the best available information from industrial experience, from experiments involving humans and other animals, and, when possible, from a combination of these. The basis on which the values are established may differ from substance to substance. Protection against impairment of health may be a guiding factor for some, whereas reasonable freedom from irritation, narcosis, nuisance, or other forms of stress may be the basis for others.

But TLVs do not always represent valid thresholds for adverse effects on health. A small percentage of workers, because of age, genetic factors, personal habits (such as cigarette smoking or the use of alcohol or other drugs), medication, or previous exposures, may experience adverse health effects from some substances at concentrations at or below the threshold limit. In most cases, maintaining exposures below the threshold should provide protection. But if the relationship between exposures (or dose) and the associated health effects is linear, there will be some effect, however small the exposure (Figure 3.1). For this reason, TLVs cannot be considered the final word on the line between safe and dangerous concentrations, nor should they be used as a definitive index of the relative toxicity of various substances. The degree of protection required by individual workers should always be evaluated by a professionally trained occupational health physician (ACGIH, 1990).

Control of Occupational Exposures

There is a wide range of occupational health problems, and each requires a different control approach. The two basic types of problems are those arising from toxic chemicals and those arising from physical factors.

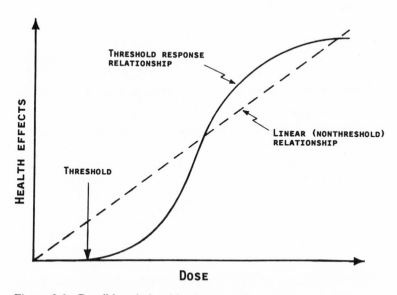

Figure 3.1 Possible relationships between dose and health effects

Toxic Chemicals

The primary problem associated with toxic chemicals is airborne contamination. Examples include releases of trichloroethylene in degreasing operations; gases and metal fumes in welding; silica dust, metal fumes, and carbon monoxide in foundries; and carbon monoxide from internal combustion engines in a variety of working environments (Burgess, 1981).

A complete and effective control program requires process and workplace monitoring systems and the education and commitment of both workers and management to good occupational health practices. All systems for controlling airborne contaminants should be designed to provide protection not only under normal operating conditions but also under conditions of process upset or failure (Gideon et al., 1979).

There are six basic approaches to controlling toxic airborne chemicals. The first four involve controlling the chemical at its source by preventing it from gaining access to the working environment. The last two are designed for situations in which the first four approaches have failed or cannot be used. In these cases the airborne toxic chemicals must be assumed to be present in the working environment.

Elimination or Substitution

This approach involves control at the source by completely eliminating use of a toxic substance or substituting a less toxic one. Examples include discontinuing the use of mercury in Leclanche type batteries and using toluene or xylene instead of the more toxic benzene in paint strippers.

Process or Equipment Modification

Another way to control hazards at the source is to modify older processes that do not meet existing or proposed occupational health standards. In general, processes that are continuous are less hazardous to workers than intermittent or batch processes. Processes should be designed to contain hazardous materials within sealed or enclosed equipment as far as practical, and to minimize maintenance requirements and associated exposures. In many cases, changes in process chemistry can minimize unwanted by-products. For example, changes in formulating a relatively nontoxic dinitroanaline herbicide have reduced by-product nitrosamines by a factor of 100. Another example of process modification is the use of robots in paint-spraying and welding operations.

Isolation or Enclosure

Operations involving highly toxic materials can be isolated from other parts of the facility by construction of a barrier between the source of the hazard and workers who might be affected. The barrier can be a physical structure or a pressure differential. A common approach is to place toxic or radioactive materials in an enclosure having a negative pressure, or to have the space occupied by workers be at a positive pressure. An example of the latter is the control room provided for operators at nuclear power plants.

Local Exhaust Ventilation or Air Cleaning

Airborne gases or particulates produced by essentially all industrial operations can be captured at their point of generation by use of an exhaust ventilation system. Success depends on a sufficient airflow to capture the contaminants as they are released and to prevent their gaining access to the working environment. Two types of equipment that can be used to do this are a glove box (Figure 3.2) and a laboratory hood (Figure 3.3).

Another strategy is to use air-cleaning devices such as filters, adsorbers, and electrostatic precipitators. However, such devices are more commonly used to remove contaminants from airstreams being discharged into the environment, for example, from local exhaust systems, rather than to clean air that is to be recirculated in the workplace. This approach is limited to the control of relatively nontoxic materials.

Personal Protective Equipment

Controls can also be applied to individual workers. In general, however, this strategy should be considered a last resort, to be used only if controls at the source or the workplace are not practical or have failed, for it can lead to a reduced emphasis on keeping the workplace free of contamination.

This approach isolates the worker rather than the source of expo-

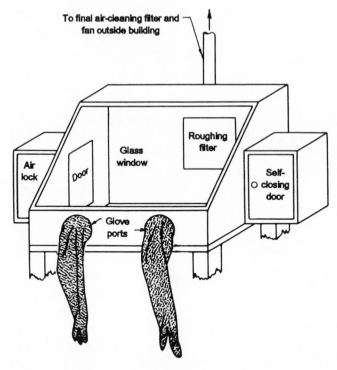

To final air-cleaning filter and
fan outside building

Roughing
filter

Glass
window

Air
lock

Door

Self-
closing
door

Glove
ports

Figure 3.2   Glove box for handling highly toxic or radioactive materials

sure from the surrounding work environment. Examples include the use of protective clothing and devices such as respirators (Figure 3.4). The choice of protective clothing should be based on the exposure hazard, the amount of body coverage required, and the material's impermeability to the hazardous agent. Because such protective garments are designed to be impervious, and thus hamper heat loss through evaporation, workers wearing them are frequently subject to heat stress.

A respirator passes air that is to be breathed by the wearer through an air-purifying element, either a filter (to remove particulates) or a sorbent (to remove gases and vapors). Because of their many disadvantages, respirators should be used only for short-term exposures or for emergency situations. These disadvantages include (1) the ever-present risk that they may fail to operate as designed; (2) limitations on the length of time that a filter or sorbent will provide adequate

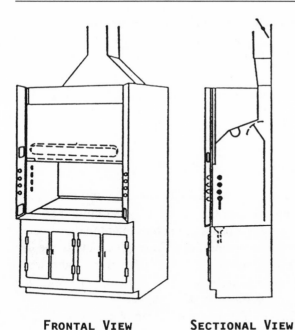

FRONTAL VIEW　　SECTIONAL VIEW

Figure 3.3　Typical laboratory hood for handling toxic chemical or radioactive materials

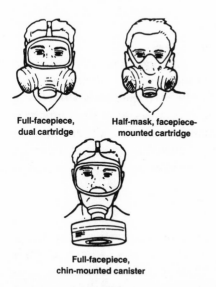

Full-facepiece,
dual cartridge

Half-mask, facepiece-
mounted cartridge

Full-facepiece,
chin-mounted canister

Figure 3.4　Several types of respirators used to protect workers from airborne contaminants

protection; (3) the difficulty of breathing through the system; (4) the accompanying discomfort, including skin irritation; (5) the high cost of maintenance (including cleaning and sterilizing); and (6) the provision, in many cases, of less protection than is assumed (which gives both the worker and the employer a false sense of security). Use of respirators may also tend to delay the installation of more effective engineering controls.

Good Work Practices and Housekeeping

Good work practices and good housekeeping are also important control strategies. Good work practices begin with proper equipment design and with structuring standard operating and maintenance procedures to minimize exposures and emissions. Examples include the use of hand-held quick-response instruments to conduct periodic leak-detection surveys, the requirement that safe-work permits be obtained before a task is begun, and the use of "lockout" systems, which prevent operation of a facility (through some form of a locking device) except when conditions are safe. Examples of good housekeeping practices are chemical decontamination, wet sweeping, and vacuuming.

Physical Factors

Physical factors in the workplace such as high temperatures, high humidity, noise, repetitive motions, vibration, and ionizing and non-ionizing radiation (discussed in Chapter 9) have specific health effects and require control techniques different from those needed for toxic chemicals. These techniques must take into account the human/machine interface and promote the use of industrial equipment designed to reduce both physical stresses and accidents.

High Temperatures or Humidity

Heat stress is a common occupational problem, particularly among workers who wear protective clothing. NIOSH has estimated that it affects as many as 6 million U.S. workers (Grubb, 1990).

As body temperature rises, the circulatory system seeks to cool the body by increasing the heart's pumping rate, dilating the blood vessels, and increasing blood flow to the skin. If these mechanisms do not provide sufficient cooling, the body will perspire, and the evaporation of sweat will cool the skin and the blood and reduce body temperature. Because sweating causes a loss of both water and electrolytes, some form of heat stress, including heat stroke, may develop if body temperature is not decreased.

The degree to which heat affects workers depends on their level of physical activity, the ventilation rate, and the relative humidity (which influences the effectiveness of perspiration as a mechanism for cooling the body). Control measures include reducing humidity to improve evaporative cooling, increasing air movement by means of natural and mechanical ventilation, providing radiant-reflecting shields between workers and the heat source, reducing work-load demands, or a combination of these. Employees should be trained both to recognize the symptoms of heat stress and to provide treatment. Such training should include a review of measures for acclimatization, fluid replacement, control of work rate, and workplace monitoring.

Noise

Noise, defined as unwanted or objectionable sound, has been one of the most common occupational problems since the Industrial Revolution. Because noise-induced hearing loss occurs gradually, invisibly, and often painlessly, many employers and employees do not recognize the problem early enough to provide protection; indeed, for years hearing loss was considered a "normal" hazard of employment. In 1989 7–10 million people in the United States worked at sites where the noise level presented some risk of hearing loss. Of the workers exposed, about 1.6 million may already have a mild hearing loss, 1.1 million a measurable hearing loss, and 0.5 million a moderate to severe hearing loss (National Safety Council, 1989). Today, compensation payments to U.S. workers for hearing losses approach $100 million per year. In addition to its obvious effects on hearing, excessive noise may affect the cardiovascular and nervous systems.

The OSHA Noise Standard requires employers to provide a hearing-conservation program, noise monitoring, hearing protection, and annual audiograms for employees whose daily exposures exceed 85 decibels, based on an 8-hour time-weighted average. Employers must also provide feasible engineering controls, require hearing pro-

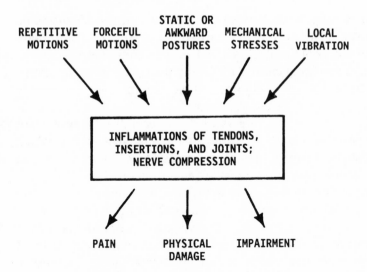

Figure 3.5   Sources and effects of physical factors in the occupational
environment

tection, or both in areas with daily exposures in excess of certain
values (OSHA, 1983). As with various airborne contaminants, noise
can be controlled at the source, by damping, reducing, or enclosing
the vibrating surface that produces it. Examples include substituting
low-speed, high-pitch fan blades for high-speed, low-pitch ones, placing sound absorbers between the source and employees, and providing hearing protection to individual workers. Like respirators,
hearing-protection devices for individuals should be considered a last
resort.

The Human/Machine Interface

Many health and safety problems in the workplace are caused by
physical stresses imposed on workers by improperly designed equipment. Such stresses include repetitive motions, forceful motions,
static or awkward postures, mechanical stresses, and local vibration
(Figure 3.5). All can lead to pain and physical damage. Reducing
these stresses often involves redesigning equipment to conform with
principles of ergonomics or human-factors engineering. Ergonomics
is increasingly being recognized as an important way to prevent both

chronic injuries and major accidents. For example, studies following the accident at the nuclear power plant at Three Mile Island in Pennsylvania showed that much of the information the operators needed if they were to understand fully the status of the plant was not readily accessible. Likewise, many aircraft accidents have been traced to instruments that could be misinterpreted, especially under conditions of stress.

Two important occupational health problems that are being addressed through human-factors engineering are low-back pain and cumulative trauma disorders. Studies show that 25 percent of all injuries in the workplace occur in the process of lifting and moving objects. Another 15–20 percent of workplace injuries occur as a result of slips and falls. Thus, these two categories represent almost half of all injuries in the workplace. The data also indicate that if a worker who has suffered a low-back injury has not returned to work within six months, he or she will probably never return (Snook, 1989).

Strategies for significantly reducing the occurrence of low-back pain among workers include the use of mechanical aids to lift heavy weights, good workplace layout (to help workers avoid unnecessary twisting and reaching), good seat design (to provide adjustment and lumbar support), and appropriate packaging of products (to match package weights with human capabilities). Similarly, designs are available for safe stairs, floors, and working surfaces.

The General Outlook

Technologies are already available for controlling many occupational health problems. Nonetheless, occupational health specialists must be alert to the multitude of changes occurring in the workplace, many of which are introducing new kinds of health problems. The U.S. work force contains an increasing number of women and minorities, is growing older as a whole, and faces ever-stronger competition from overseas production, which may lessen resolve to maintain high occupational health standards. An increasingly complex array of materials, new processes, and equipment is being used in industrial operations. Today many workplace hazards are less obvious and less clearly related to the job. These hazards include effects on the reproductive system and a host of subtle injuries, diseases, and disabilities resulting from low-level on-the-job psychological stress. Our ability to assess the effects of these changes on occupational health will require input from a wide range of specialists including social and behavioral scientists, public health research workers, medical care specialists, and many others who may currently view the problems of occupational health as being outside their profession (Walker, 1988).

As a result of these changes, the success or failure of occupational health programs depends heavily on corporate leaders' awareness that changes are occurring in workers' attitudes and needs; that provision of a safe workplace is increasingly important; and that occupational health program decisions have long-term economic impacts. In fact improvements in the health of the work force often depend more on changes in the values of corporate management than on technical considerations. Fortunately, many corporate leaders are now beginning to emphasize the role of physical activity, nutrition programs, stress management, and other healthy lifestyle behaviors in the health and productivity of the work force.

The U.S. Department of Health and Human Services (1990) has recognized the importance of a safe and healthy occupational environment in its *National Health Goals for the Year 2000*. Areas that have been targeted for improvement include (1) increasing to 70 percent the number of smaller worksites (fewer than 50 workers) with health and safety programs, (2) increasing to 80 percent the number of larger worksites (more than 750 workers) with employer-sponsored opportunities for physical activity, and (3) achieving an across-the-board reduction in repetitive-motion disorders and work-related injuries. Experience has shown that proactive programs related to areas such as improved physical fitness, alcohol abuse, and injury prevention yield as much as a four-to-one economic benefit to employers through reduced employee turnover, illness, and absenteeism.

REFERENCES

ACGIH. 1990. *1990–1991 Threshold Limit Values for Chemical Substances and Physical Agents and Biological Exposure Indices*. Cincinnati.

Burgess, William A. 1981. *Recognition of Health Hazards in Industry*. New York: Wiley-Interscience.

Corn, M. 1989. "The Progression of Industrial Hygiene." *Applied Industrial Hygiene* 4, no. 6 (June), 153–157.

Cralley, Lewis, and Walter H. Konn. 1973. "The Significance and Uses of Guides, Codes, Regulations, and Standards for Chemical and Physical Agents." In *The Industrial Environment: Its Evaluation & Control.* Washington, D.C.: U.S. Department of Health, Education and Welfare.

Gideon, J. A., E. R. Kennedy, D. M. O'Brien, and J. T. Talty. 1979. *Controlling Occupational Exposures: Principles and Practices.* Cincinnati: National Institute for Occupational Safety and Health, U.S. Department of Health, Education and Welfare.

Grubb, Gregg. 1990. "Occupational Health—More than Just Asbestos." *ECON: Environmental Contractor* 5, no. 7 (July), 50–53.

Hamilton, Alice. 1943. *Exploring the Dangerous Trades.* Boston: Little, Brown.

National Safety Council. 1989. *Accident Facts, 1989 Edition.* Chicago.

———. 1990. *Accident Facts, 1990 Edition.* Chicago.

OSHA. 1983. "Occupational Noise Exposure: Hearing Conservation Amendment." *Federal Register* 48, no. 46 (8 March), 9738–83.

Patty, F. A. 1978. "Industrial Hygiene: Retrospect and Prospect." In *Patty's Industrial Hygiene and Toxicology,* ed. G. D. Clayton and F. E. Clayton. Vol. 1. 3d rev. ed. New York: John Wiley and Sons.

Snook, S. H. 1989. "The Control of Low Back Disability: The Role of Management." *In Manual Material Handling: Understanding and Preventing Back Trauma,* ed. K. H. E. Kroemer, J. D. McGlothlin, and T. G. Bobick. Akron: American Industrial Hygiene Association.

U.S. Department of Health and Human Services. 1990. *National Health Goals for the Year 2000.* Washington, D.C.

Walker, Bailus. 1988. "President's Column." *Nation's Health,* August, p. 2.

Weiss, Bernard. 1990. "Neurotoxic Risks in the Workplace." *Applied Occupational and Environmental Hygiene* 6, no. 9 (September), 587–594.

4

Water and Sewage

Approximately 70 percent of the earth is covered by water, but only 3 percent is not salty and is therefore potentially available for consumption by plants and animals. Of this 3 percent, about two-thirds is frozen in the polar icecaps and in glaciers and is therefore unavailable. Another 0.7 percent is below the earth's surface, as groundwater, and only a small fraction is close enough to the surface to be readily accessible for human use. About 0.3 percent of the fresh water is available as surface sources. Thus, well under 1 percent of the water on earth is available for human use (UNESCO, 1971). However, this volume totals several hundred thousand cubic miles (10^{15} cubic meters) (Chanlett, 1979). The volume of groundwater in the upper one-half mile of the earth's crust in the contiguous 48 states is estimated to be 50,000 cubic miles (Council on Environmental Quality, 1989).

The basic source of all water on earth is precipitation—rain, snow, and sleet. Of the precipitation reaching the earth's surface, however, only about 30 percent falls on land areas, and that is not evenly distributed. Average annual precipitation in the United States is about 30 inches per year; however, the range varies from a few tenths of an inch in the desert areas of the Southwest to 400 inches or more in some parts of Hawaii. About 40 percent of the contiguous United States (primarily areas east of the Mississippi River) receives over 75 percent of the rainfall (Council on Environmental Quality, 1989). Worldwide, the distribution of rainfall is still more uneven. In any given year, departures from average conditions can be extreme.

About 70 percent of the precipitation that reaches land areas is evaporated or transpired (through vegetation) directly back into the atmosphere; 10 percent soaks in and becomes groundwater, and 20 percent runs off into lakes, streams, and rivers. Most of this surface

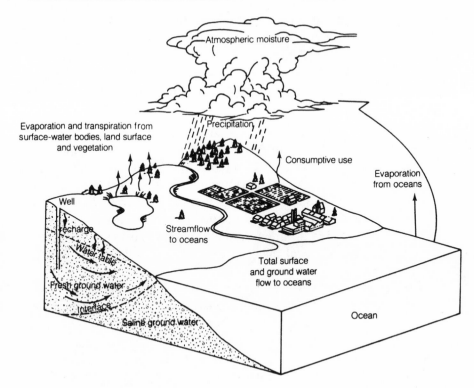

Figure 4.1   The hydrologic cycle

and ground water ultimately flows into the oceans. The overall movement of water from precipitation through various pathways on earth and back into the atmosphere is called the hydrologic cycle (Figure 4.1).

Human Uses of Water

People in the developed nations use water for a wide variety of purposes, many of them indirect or almost unnoticed, and most of them wasteful. In 1985 almost 400 billion gallons of water per day were withdrawn from aquifers and streams in the United States for public water supply, rural use, irrigation, and industry. Of this amount, 307 billion gallons were eventually discharged into rivers and streams, and 92 billion gallons were consumed and incorporated into manufactured products, agricultural crops, and animal tissue and hence were no longer available for immediate use. Direct human consumption accounts for only about 3 percent of all water used; water that meets drinking-water standards is also routinely used for irrigating lawns, fighting fires, washing cars, cleaning streets, and recreational and aesthetic purposes.

Personal use: Personal uses include drinking, cooking, bathing, laundering, and excreta disposal. On a daily basis, flushing the toilet consumes some 15–25 gallons (60–90 liters), drinking and cooking about 2 quarts (2 liters), and bathing about 15–20 gallons.

Waste carriage: The water-carriage method of excreta disposal, an outgrowth of the development of the flush toilet, uses 250 gallons of water, purified at an enormous economic cost, to transport a single pound of fecal material to a sewage treatment plant for disposal.

Recreational and aesthetic uses: These uses include swimming, boating, sailing, water skiing, fountains, and the like. Except for discharges of oil and gasoline from power boats into lakes and rivers, few of these uses result in significant pollution.

Irrigation: About 140 billion gallons of water are used each day in the United States for irrigation. About half of this comes from surface water and half from groundwater sources. In the years 1940–1985 the use of water for irrigation in the United States doubled, and over the past three decades the removal of groundwater for this purpose has increased even faster (Council on Environmental Quality, 1989). The use of groundwater for irrigation is highest in the western states—Arizona, California, Idaho, Kansas, Nebraska, and Texas. In contrast to most other uses, irrigation water is no longer available for direct reuse: whereas water used by humans for other purposes is either excreted or returned to the earth, most water taken up by plants is transpired into the atmosphere.

Other uses: Other uses of water include aquaculture, transportation (waterways and canals), and the generation of power (hydroelectric power plants).

Few people in industrialized nations are aware of the many ways in which water is used in support of their accepted standard of living. Consider the following examples: It is estimated that more than 50 glasses of water are required to grow the oranges necessary to provide one glass of orange juice (Anonymous, 1991). About 120 gallons of water are required to produce one chicken egg (this includes the water required to grow a chicken to the age at which she can lay eggs and to feed her subsequently); about 3,500 gallons are required to produce a steak; and about 60,000 gallons are required to produce one ton of steel (roughly the amount required for an automobile) (Canby, 1980).

Today efforts are under way worldwide to reduce the quantity of water used for various daily activities. These include the development of toilets that can be flushed with much smaller amounts of water, and of faucets and showerheads that can operate at reduced rates of flow; the recycling of treated sewage for use in industrial processes; improved methods of irrigation ("drip irrigation") to deliver water directly to the plants; and the use of treated sewage (rather than drinking water) to irrigate recreational areas such as golf courses. Table 4.1 presents the amounts of water that can be saved through the use of water-efficient household fixtures. Congress is considering bills that would mandate limits on the water consumption of various household devices, such as dish and clothes washers. These requirements would parallel those imposed on the energy efficiency of other household products such as hot-water heaters, refrigerators, and furnaces.

Sources of Drinking Water

There are three primary sources of drinking water. Each has its advantages and disadvantages.

Groundwater

The widespread use of groundwater stems not only from its general availability but also from economic and public health considerations. Groundwater is commonly available at the point of need at relatively little cost, and its use does not require the construction of reservoirs and long pipelines. It is normally free of suspended solids, bacteria, and other disease-causing organisms, so it does not require extensive treatment except in limited areas where it has been polluted (Council on Environmental Quality, 1989). It can be obtained through bored, driven, or drilled wells and through collection from springs that flow to the surface.

Table 4.1   Potential water savings from using water-efficient
instead of conventional household systems

System	Water consumption		Savings (%)
	Gallons	Liters	
Toilets[a]			
Conventional	5	19	
Common low-flush	3.5	13	32
Washdown	1	4	79
Air assisted	0.5	2	89
Clothes washers[a]			
Conventional	37	140	
Wash recycle	26	100	29
Front loading	21	80	43
Showerheads[b]			
Conventional	5	19	
Common low-flow	3	11	42
Flow limiting	2	7	63
Air assisted	0.5	2	89
Faucets[b]			
Conventional	3	12	
Common low-flow	2.5	10	17
Flow limiting	1.5	6	50

a. Consumption per use.
b. Consumption per minute.

Accessible groundwater sources are limited in volume and, once depleted, are essentially irreplaceable. Withdrawal at too rapid a rate can cause major disruption of land areas: some areas in Texas and California have subsided as much as 1–2 meters and in Mexico City as much as 10 meters; low-lying areas have become vulnerable to flooding. In Florida some land areas have collapsed, and in certain coastal areas withdrawals have so depleted the volume of fresh water that salty ocean water has moved in to take its place. To correct this situation, several states are diverting rainfall to holding ponds to encourage the water to seep back into the ground and recharge the local aquifers.

Protected Runoff

Some cities (such as New York, Boston, and Lisbon) establish protected watersheds, collect the precipitation that falls on them, and use that as their drinking-water supply. The water is disinfected (usually by chlorination) before use. Similarly, an individual household may collect the rain falling on the roof of a house and store it in a cistern for use as needed. Such supplies are generally used without treatment.

One major problem with these sources is that, because of the presence of many chemicals in the atmosphere, rainfall is no longer pure. Acid rain, if it falls directly on the ground, dissolves minerals from the soil and carries them into lakes and streams. Another problem is that it is becoming increasingly difficult to establish new protected (uninhabited) land areas to use for the collection of drinking-water supplies. In addition, the presence of growths of aquatic organisms, such as algae, in reservoirs frequently produces unacceptably bad tastes and odors when the supplies are chlorinated for human consumption.

Surface Supplies

Lakes, streams, and rivers serve as sources of water for many cities. Such sources, however, usually require extensive treatment (purification) before use, and industrial pollution has increased the costs of purification. There is also concern in many parts of the world about the adequacy of surface water supplies (especially where there is also local demand for irrigation).

Health Hazards from Drinking Water

In the developed nations, the introduction of disinfection practices shortly after 1900 virtually eliminated many infectious diseases that are transmitted through the ingestion of water. Today, however, concern is growing about the health implications of a host of other contaminants, particularly toxic chemicals. Evaluations of their health effects are complicated by the same problems faced in essentially all other fields of environmental and occupational health, namely, the latency (time delay) in the appearance of the effects and the lack of definitive data on dose-response relationships. In addition, the federal government has been slow to acknowledge the importance of drinking water to health: the first federal legislation directly addressing the subject, the Safe Water Drinking Act, was not passed until December 1974.

One of the first scientists to examine the possible role of drinking water in health was H. A. Schroeder of Dartmouth College, who demonstrated what appeared to be a clear correlation between heart disease and the "hardness," or mineral content, of water (Schroeder, 1974). He found that people who drank "soft" water (containing few minerals) had a higher incidence of heart disease, apparently because soft water, being corrosive, dissolves toxic substances (such as lead, cadmium, and other harmful chemicals) from plumbing systems before being ingested. Schroeder's studies have been expanded by others, notably by the National Institute of Environmental Health Sciences and the EPA. An excellent reference is the National Research Council's nine-volume *Drinking Water and Health* (1977–1989).

Water Supplies and Purification

Preparing water for human consumption is a major industry. There are about 60,000 municipal water purification and distribution systems in the United States alone. Of these, about 11,000 use surface water supplies, providing drinking water to about 150 million people; those using groundwater supplies serve about 100 million. The combined output of these systems is 40–50 billion gallons per day, or 160–200 gallons for each person in the United States. Fifty-seven percent of this is used domestically, 32 percent is used by commercial groups and industry, 9 percent is used for public services (fighting fires, cleaning streets, watering parks), and 2 percent is lost through leaks in the distribution system (U.S. Geological Survey, 1988). In addition, many industries have their own purification systems. Most water used for irrigation is taken directly from rivers, lakes, or the ground and used without prior treatment.

The capital investment in municipal water treatment facilities totals about $250 billion, and the annual cost of operating them is about $5 billion. The low cost of drinking water (still well under a dollar per ton) does not reflect the true cost of producing the water or the fact that many sources currently being used, particularly those underground, will be depleted within the next few decades. As more and more contaminants gain access to surface and groundwater, the cost of purifying and distributing water can be expected to increase substantially.

The primary purposes of a water purification or treatment system are to collect water from a source of supply, purify it for drinking if necessary, and distribute it to consumers. Since most groundwater sources do not require treatment, the following discussion focuses on the two principal methods of purifying surface water supplies: slow sand filtration and rapid sand filtration.

Slow Sand Filtration

In this relatively simple process, the raw water supply is passed slowly through a sand bed 2–3 feet (60–90 centimeters) deep. Soon after a bed is placed in operation, a biological growth develops on top and within the sand, removing and retaining particles from the raw water. This process removes most bacteria and disease organisms, including the cysts of *Giardia lamblia,* the organism that causes giardiasis (Chapter 5). Because excess turbidity in the raw water supply will rapidly plug the filter bed, preliminary settling is recommended. A filter bed area of 2,000 square feet (185 square meters) will provide approximately 100,000 gallons of treated water per day. With proper care, filter beds can be operated 30–200 days before the top layers of sand have to be scraped, cleaned, or replaced. In other respects such systems require minimal maintenance (Allen et al., 1988; Leland and Damewood, 1990).

Rapid Sand Filtration

Figure 4.2 shows the principal steps in this process, described below.

Raw Water Storage

Water is pumped or diverted from a river or stream into a raw water storage basin. Such storage provides a carryover or reserve in case the raw water supply becomes unfit for use for several days, say, through the accidental release of a contaminant upstream of the supply. Storage also removes color and reduces turbidity and bacteria.

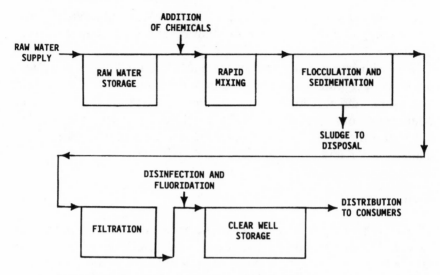

Figure 4.2   Principal steps in the water purification process

Addition of Chemicals, Rapid Mixing, and Coagulation

Chemicals are added to the water to create a coagulant. The chemical most commonly used in the United States is $Al_2(SO_4)_3 \cdot 14H_2O$, commonly called alum. A less frequently used chemical is ferric chloride ($FeCl_3$). The basic reactions produced are almost identical:

$$Al^{+++} + 3HCO_3^- \rightarrow Al(OH)_3 + 3CO_2$$

and

$$Fe^{+++} + 3HCO_3^- \rightarrow Fe(OH)_3 + 3CO_2.$$

The highly positively charged Al^{+++} and Fe^{+++} ions also attract the negatively charged colloidal suspended matter in the water and together with the $Al(OH)_3$ or $Fe(OH)_3$ form a gelatinous mass called floc. Rapid mixing is essential to provide maximum interaction between the positive metallic ions and the negative colloidal suspended matter.

Although theoretically a good chemist could calculate the proper amount of alum or ferric chloride to add to the raw water for optimum coagulation and flocculation, this quantity is most commonly determined on the basis of a jar test. This consists of adding a known amount of water to a series of jars or beakers, adding a different concentration of coagulant to each, and then observing which concentration (dosage) coagulates and flocculates best. This dosage is then used for the full-scale operation. Since the characteristics of the water supply are subject to change, jar tests are generally conducted at least once a day.

Flocculation and Sedimentation

Once coagulation has been accomplished by the rapid mixing, the water is slowly and gently stirred to enable the finely divided floc to agglomerate into larger particles that will rapidly settle. This process, called flocculation, is accomplished by moving large paddles slowly and gently through the water. Since water treatment is performed as a continuous flow-through process, flocculation often takes place as the water enters one end of a large tank, with settling of the floc (sedimentation) taking place at the other end. During flocculation, larger particles in the water (including bacteria) are enmeshed in the floc, and ionic, colloidal, and suspended particles are adsorbed on its surface. This process, however, removes no contaminants that may be dissolved in the water (Chanlett, 1979).

For sedimentation, the water is allowed to undergo a period of quiescence. The settled floc or sludge is removed from the bottom of the settling tank and sent to disposal. Originally, such settling was accomplished in a large rectangular tank and required a quiescent period of 2–4 hours. More recently, high-rate-settling tanks have been developed in which the water is passed through small-diameter tubes (or between parallel plates) set at an angle within a larger tank (Montgomery, 1985). Because the solids in the water have to travel a shorter distance before reaching a surface on which to deposit, and because this arrangement provides unique flow conditions, the required detention time for clarifying the water is only about 20 minutes. This approach also significantly reduces the required settling-tank space.

Filtration

Because the settled water will still retain some traces of floc, it is passed through a bed of sand 2–3 feet deep. Such beds, which use a combination of adsorption, additional flocculation and sedimentation, and straining, remove even the smallest particles (Chanlett, 1979).

Sand filters become loaded with floc and must be cleaned by backwashing with purified drinking water every 12–72 hours. The waste water is sent to the sewer. About 2 percent of the water produced in a water purification facility is required for backwashing.

Disinfection and Fluoridation

Once the clarified water is disinfected and fluoride added for the prevention of dental caries, it is sent to clear well storage and is ready for distribution to consumers. If chlorine is used as a disinfectant, usually a slight excess is added so that a small residual will accompany the water entering the distribution system. This strategy protects consumers in case bacterial contaminants later somehow gain access to the water. Chlorine, however, often produces unwanted tastes and odors in water, particularly if certain forms of microscopic algae are present. If the water contains organic contaminants, the addition of chlorine will produce chlorinated hydrocarbons, which are known to be carcinogenic. Chlorinated hydrocarbons are also volatile, so they are readily released into the air when water is used in dish and clothes washers, in showers, and in flushing a toilet (McKone, 1987).

There are three ways to prevent the production of chlorinated hydrocarbons:

1. The water can be chlorinated for several minutes to kill the viruses and bacteria, and then immediately dechlorinated by the addition of sulfur dioxide or ammonia.
2. Instead of chlorine, ozone can be used as a disinfectant. However, ozone is expensive and does not maintain a residual. To provide a disinfection residual in the water distribution system, a small amount of chlorine can be added to the water immediately before distribution.
3. The water can be treated with chlorine and then aerated to remove the chlorinated hydrocarbons. Care must be taken, however, that people are not exposed to the airborne releases.

Table 4.2 summarizes the effects of various steps in the water purification process on specific characteristics of the raw water supply.

Variations in the basic processes described above include proce-

Table 4.2 Effects of purification processes on specific characteristics of water

Process	Characteristic						
	Bacterial content	Color	Turbidity	Taste and odor	Hardness (calcium and magnesium)	Corrosiveness	Iron and manganese
Raw water storage	+	+	+	±	+	0	+
Aeration	0	0	0	+	0	+	+
Coagulation and sedimentation	+	+	+	0	0	−	+
Lime-soda softening	+	0	+	0	+	+	+
Sand filtration	+	+	+	0	0	0	+
Chlorination or ozonation	+	+	0	±	0	0	+
Carbon adsorption	−	+	+	+	0	0	0

Note: 0 = no effect; + = beneficial effect (aids in alleviating the problem); − = negative effect (adds to the problem); ± = sometimes beneficial, sometimes negative effect.

dures to remove hardness, iron and manganese, organic compounds, and tastes and odors.

Removal of Hardness

To remove hardness from small volumes of water, such as for an individual household, the ion-exchange process is generally used. The lime-soda process tends to be used for large volumes. In the latter process, calcium hydroxide (lime) and sodium carbonate are added to the water and interact with dissolved calcium (hardness) to form insoluble calcium carbonate, which precipitates and thus reduces the concentration of calcium.

Removal of Iron and Manganese

Iron and manganese are soluble in water only in the reduced chemical state. If oxidized, they immediately become insoluble and precipitate. Thus they are readily removed from water by aeration.

Control of Organic Compounds, and Tastes, and Odors

One of the best methods for removing organic compounds (and similar chemicals that produce unwanted tastes and odors) from water is to adsorb them on activated carbon (charcoal). If concentrations of the organic compounds are low, activated carbon (available in powder form) can be placed on top of the sand filter or mixed with the chemical coagulants. If concentrations of organic compounds in the raw water supply are relatively high, the preferred approach is to place the carbon in an adsorption bed separate from the sand filter. To be effective, the bed must provide up to 15 minutes of contact between the carbon and the water. Often this requires a bed as much as 9 feet deep. Such a bed will last from 6 weeks to 6 months, depending on the concentration of organic compounds in the water.

Despite the care with which water supplies of major municipalities are prepared, trace elements and contaminants may remain in the treated water and may have an effect on health. Improved methods for water purification are constantly being developed.

Excreta Disposal and Sewage Treatment

Methods for disposing of human excreta have evolved from very simple approaches, such as the pit privy, to the major water-carriage systems of today. Not all these changes amount to improvements, particularly from the standpoint of conservation of resources.

One of the earliest and simplest methods for disposing of human excreta was the pit privy, a hole in the ground with a small closed shelter and toilet built above it. Generally the hole is about 3 feet in diameter and about 6 feet deep. An essential part of an effective privy is a screen-covered vent pipe, which provides a natural pathway for removing odors and for trapping flies and other insects. Privy designs range from those in which excreta are deposited on the surface of the ground to those in which excreta are collected in a bucket or tank for later removal and disposal elsewhere. Double-vault privies are used by many people in the developing countries. Switching pits once a year provides sufficient retention and decomposition to assure the destruction of most pathogenic organisms.

With the development of the water closet or flush toilet, sewage treatment and disposal entered a new era. Although the Minoans in Crete in 2800 B.C. had toilets that could be flushed either with rainwater or with water stored in cisterns, the invention of the modern flush toilet is generally credited to Sir John Harrington in 1596 (Chanlett, 1979). Queen Elizabeth I admired the concept and had one built for her own use, but the idea had to wait until the eighteenth century for further development. In 1775 Alexander Cummings patented a water closet with a valve for initiating the flush and a trap to seal off odors. However, the valve controlling the inflow of water allowed considerable leakage. This problem was solved by Sir Thomas Crapper, who in 1872 invented the first valveless water waste preventer. The principles of his design continue in use today. By the early 1800s most wealthy people had at least one water closet that discharged either onto the ground or into a cesspool, an underground pit. Thomas Jefferson had a water closet installed in the White House in 1800. In 1855 George Vanderbilt had the first bathroom (consisting of a lavatory, porcelain tub, and flush toilet) built inside an American house. As late as the 1880s, however, only one of every six people in U.S. cities had access to modern bathroom facilities.

Individual Household Disposal

With the advent of the flush toilet, methods had to be developed for disposing of the discharged wastes. Most municipalities have constructed systems that carry the effluent to a sewer and then to some form of municipal sewage treatment plant. However, some 30–35 percent of the U.S. population, or 75–90 million people, are not served by sewers. They depend instead on some form of on-site subsurface sewage disposal system. The most common of these is the septic tank.

Septic Tank

A septic tank is usually constructed of concrete, with an inlet and an outlet for sewage to enter and leave (Figure 4.3). As sewage passes through the tank, solids settle to the bottom and undergo anaerobic digestion. Most tanks have a divider in the bottom and a baffle at the top near the outlet end to help prevent carryover of settled solids and floating material in the effluent. Under proper operating conditions, the effluent is clear and is discharged into a drain field consisting of open-jointed or perforated pipe through which the liquid can seep into the surrounding soil. For proper performance, it is generally recommended that (1) the tank have a volume of at least 500 gallons, (2) the soil in which the drain field is located be sufficiently porous to absorb the liquid effluent, (3) the land area be adequate for complete adsorption of the effluent flow, and (4) the tank be cleaned (the solids removed) every few years.

The last recommendation is extremely important because if solids are permitted to build up too long in the tank they will be carried out with the effluent and will seal up the drain field.

Only about one-third of the soils in the United States are suitable for adsorbing septic tank effluents. About 25 percent of the tanks malfunction either periodically or continually because they have been installed improperly or in unsuitable soils. Under these conditions the effluent cannot be adsorbed and will break through to the ground surface or will find its way into a flowing groundwater source, resulting in bacterial and viral contamination of the surface soil or contamination of drinking-water supplies.

Because of the problems with septic tanks, several alternative treatment systems have been developed for the disposal of household sewage. One of these is an aerobic system. The sewage effluent is col-

Ground level

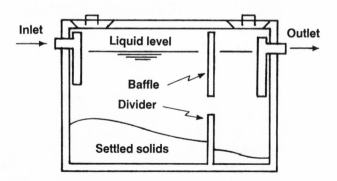

Figure 4.3   Cross-section of a typical septic tank

lected in a tank. An electric pump in the tank mixes air into the sewage to break up the solids and to accelerate the digestion process. An aerobic system is less prone than a septic tank to produce disagreeable odors, and the effluent contains dissolved oxygen, which helps prevent clogging of the drain field. One company has developed a system in which the effluent can be recycled and used for flushing the toilet again.

Other approaches include biological toilets, composting toilets, incinerating toilets, oil-flushed toilets, and vacuum disposal systems. One of the most popular of these is the Clivus Multrum household excreta and garbage disposal system, developed in Sweden. All these systems feature low water usage. The vacuum disposal systems require only about 1 quart of water per flush.

Even with improved systems for the disposal of toilet wastes, disposing of other domestic wastewater (from dish and clothes washers, bathtubs, and showers) remains a problem. However, these wastes carry fewer pathogenic organisms than the effluent from toilets. Filtration systems may be able to cleanse such water enough for use in irrigating lawns and washing cars.

Pretreatment Requirements for Industrial Waste

Municipal and industrial waste may differ significantly in composition and toxicity. In fact some kinds of industrial waste can disrupt the proper operation of municipal sewage treatment plants. For example, toxic pollutants may inhibit the growth of bacteria needed in biological treatment processes, such as the activated sludge process (discussed below), resulting in the discharge of improperly treated waste. Even if they do not interfere with treatment systems, pollutants may pass through without being adequately treated because the systems are not designed to remove them. For this reason, federal law now requires that certain industrial waste undergo treatment before being discharged into municipal sewer systems or into surface waters.

The Clean Water Act of 1977 established a system for regulating industries that discharge waste into a municipal treatment system. The act set up the National Pollutant Discharge Elimination System (NPDES) and authorized the EPA to set pretreatment standards for pollutants discharged into public waters or sewer systems that would interfere with, pass through, or otherwise be incompatible with the treatment process. Among other things, the pretreatment requirements prohibit the discharge of pollutants that create a fire or explosion hazard, are corrosive, obstruct flow in a sewer system or interfere with its operation, disrupt the treatment process, or increase the temperature of wastewater entering the treatment plant to above 104°F (40°C). To accomplish these goals, the NPDES requires all industries discharging such wastes into surface waters to install the best available control technology, and all industries discharging such wastes into municipal sewer systems must meet secondary sewage treatment standards. The EPA standards focus on toxic pollutants that are not adequately treated by municipal treatment systems. Under the NPDES, the EPA has the authority to enter and inspect industrial sources of water pollution, to sample direct and indirect discharges, and to inspect the monitoring equipment and accompanying records. Detailed regulations for enforcing this program are contained in the Code of Federal Regulations, Title 40, Parts 122–125. This program is achieving significant progress in eliminating the discharge of toxic industrial wastes both to surface waters and to municipal sewage treatment plants.

Measuring the Effectiveness of Sewage Treatment: The Biochemical Oxygen Demand (BOD) Test

Methods for treating municipal sewage are basically designed to stabilize or oxidize the organic matter in the sewage. Measuring the amount of organic matter provides an indication of how effective any treatment process is in stabilizing the sewage, and how detrimental the effect would be if the sewage were discharged into the environment.

If raw or partially treated sewage is discharged into a well-oxygenated river or stream, aerobic organisms there will begin to oxidize the organic matter biochemically. This process will remove dissolved oxygen (DO) from the stream, but eddies and other turbulence in the flowing water and the growth of green algae and other plants will add oxygen at the same time. So long as the amount of sewage is small enough in relation to the volume of the diluting water (and if additional pollution is not discharged into the same receiving body), there will always be some dissolved oxygen present. However, if oxygen is depleted faster than it is replaced, the DO concentration may become too low to support aquatic life. After reaching a minimum concentration of DO, the stream will ultimately recover. Figure 4.4 shows the "oxygen sag curve," a schematic plot of the DO concentration in a stream as a function of time or of the distance downstream from the point of sewage discharge.

The concentration of dissolved oxygen in a stream is expressed in units of milligrams of oxygen per liter of water. Since one milligram per liter represents one part of oxygen per million parts of water, oxygen concentrations in water are generally reported in terms of parts per million (ppm). The same unit is used to express the oxygen demand of sewage (that is, its potential for polluting a stream). The test most often used to assess the amount of organic matter in sewage is the Five-Day, 20°C Biochemical Oxygen Demand (BOD) test. A related chemical test has been developed to assess the oxygen demand of toxic wastes that would inhibit bacterial growth and would therefore not permit the use of a BOD test. This test is routinely used in assessing the potential polluting effects of industrial waste.

The BOD test is essentially a measure of the polluting capability or "strength" of a sewage sample; that is, it is a measure of the amount of dissolved oxygen needed to stabilize the decomposable organic matter in the waste through aerobic bacterial action. A typical BOD test is conducted in the laboratory and consists of the following steps:

1. A known percentage of sewage (usually 1–5 percent), diluted with thoroughly aerated water containing certain minerals and buffering agents, is put into two identical bottles.
2. The concentration of dissolved oxygen is measured in one of the

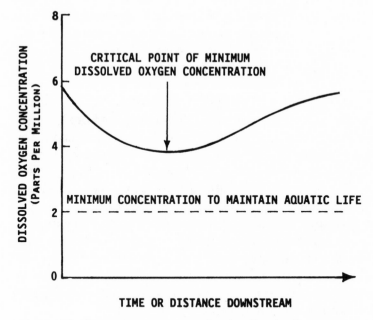

Figure 4.4   An oxygen sag curve, showing dissolved oxygen concentrations as a function of time, distance, or both in a stream into which sewage has been discharged

bottles; the second bottle is tightly sealed, placed in an incubator, and maintained at 20°C (68°F) for 5 days.

3. After 5 days the concentration of DO remaining in the second bottle is measured.
4. The difference between the DO concentrations in the bottle measured immediately and in the one measured after 5 days' incubation represents the amount of oxygen required to stabilize the sewage sample over that period. The total oxygen demand of a 100 percent sample of the sewage can be calculated on the basis of the reduction in DO concentration and the concentration of sewage originally added to the bottle.

In general, the BOD exhibited after 5 days will be approximately 70 percent of that which would be exhibited if the sample were incubated until all the organic matter in the sample was stabilized. The selection of 20°C for the BOD test is based on the fact that it is a representative outdoor temperature for a spring or fall day. At higher temperatures the BOD rate will be higher; at lower temperatures, it will be lower.

Municipal Sewage Treatment

There are three stages of treatment that can be applied to municipal sewage: primary, secondary, and tertiary. Each represents a progressive level of purification, and the number of treatment stages applied depends on the degree of treatment required. As Figure 4.5 shows, all treatment must begin with the primary stage.

Primary Treatment

Primary treatment consists in simply holding sewage in a large tank to permit the removal of solids by sedimentation. Before entering the settling tank, the sewage is commonly sent through a chamber or collector to remove sand, grit, and small rocks that would otherwise damage pumps or other equipment in the treatment plant. The settling tanks are operated on a flow-through basis and are large enough to hold the material for several hours. During that time, approximately half the solids settle out, providing a BOD reduction of 30–50 percent.

Grease and light solids that float are removed from the settling tank by a scraper and are pumped along with the settled solids to a large closed tank called a digester, where they are held for anaerobic digestion. Digestion is most effective when the sludge is heated to 90°F (32°C) or more. At 95°F the sludge is digested in about 24 days; at 130°F, in about 12 days. Methane gas produced in the process provides fuel for heating the digester.

After digestion, the sludge is stabilized and can be spread out on sand to dry in the sun. In some cases the dried sludge is used for fertilizer; in other cases it is used for landfill. Some cities, such as New York, transport digested sludge out to sea and dump it there. This approach, however, is receiving ever-closer scrutiny. The manner of disposal should not create additional public health problems. For example, sludge from urban areas may contain high concentrations of toxic chemicals (Baldwin, 1976). If the sludge is used for fertilizer, these chemicals can be taken up by food crops destined for human consumption. A notable example is cadmium, which tends to concentrate in leafy vegetables.

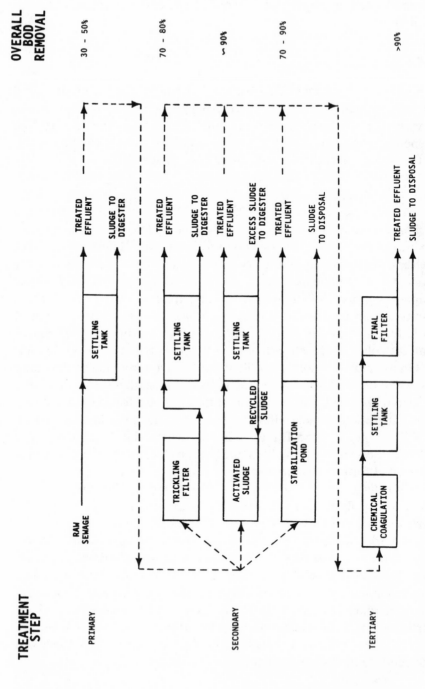

Figure 4.5 Primary, secondary, and tertiary stages in treating municipal sewage

Secondary Treatment

After primary treatment (settling), sewage can be subjected to secondary or biological treatment. In most cases this is accomplished by use of a trickling filter, an activated sludge process, or a waste stabilization pond. The first two processes are aerobic; the last combines aerobic and anaerobic systems.

TRICKLING FILTER

This is one of the most common forms of secondary treatment. The term *filter,* however, is a misnomer, since the system does not filter the sewage. Rather a trickling filter consists of a large tank, roughly 6 feet deep, filled with 2-to-4-inch stones over which sewage is intermittently trickled or sprayed from a distributor. The stones rapidly become coated with a biological film or slime. The solids in the sewage percolating through the bed are incorporated into the bacterial growth, where the microorganisms convert the organic matter into cell protoplasm and inorganic matter.

When the bacterial growth on the stones becomes too thick and heavy, it sloughs off and is carried away in the liquid effluent leaving the bottom of the filter bed. The effluent is sent to a secondary settling tank, where the bacterial sloughings settle to the bottom as a sludge. The settled effluent represents the treated product. The sludge is sent to a digester for anaerobic decomposition. The total BOD removal from a trickling filter plant is 70–80 percent. For somewhat greater BOD removals, two trickling filters can be used in series, or a single unit can be used and a portion of the settled effluent recycled through the filter bed. Figure 4.6 shows the trickling-filter treatment process.

ACTIVATED SLUDGE PROCESS

The activated sludge process is another form of aerobic secondary treatment for municipal sewage. Sewage is sent into a large open tank, where it is held for several hours and its oxygen content maintained by means of aerators (air diffusers) or mechanical agitators (paddles or brushes). Rather than growing on the surfaces of stones as in the trickling filter, the microorganisms float as suspended particles in the aerated sewage. The effluent is sent to a secondary settling tank,

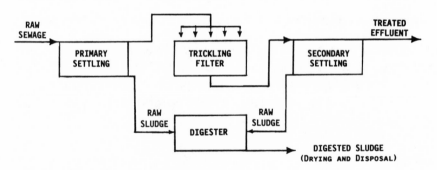

Figure 4.6 Trickling-filter sewage treatment

where the microorganisms settle out, and the settled sewage represents the treated product. BOD reductions are about 90 percent. Some of the microorganisms that have settled out in the secondary settling tank are pumped back into the aerated tank to maintain an adequate population of microbial growth. The rest of the growth is treated as sludge and sent to a digester.

WASTE STABILIZATION POND

Waste stabilization ponds have been used in other countries for many years but were largely ignored in the United States until the 1950s (Gloyna, 1971). Since then more and more have been built, particularly in the South. These simple ponds dug in the ground are typically 3–6 feet deep, 90 feet wide, and 300 feet long. They are operated on a flow-through basis and are generally designed to provide a retention time of 30–80 days. They are cheap to construct, easy to operate, and require minimal maintenance. One pond can serve 1,000–2,000 people. However, care should be taken not to locate them in soils with fissures that allow the sewage to move through the ground without filtration, thus contaminating groundwater supplies.

Waste stabilization ponds can be used singly or in series. They can be designed to receive either raw sewage or sewage that has undergone primary treatment. Most ponds operate biologically at two levels: the lower portion is anaerobic, and the upper portion is aerobic. In the border area, facultative bacteria (which can live under either aerobic or anaerobic conditions) are active. Algae growth at the surface helps assure aerobic conditions. When the pond fills with sludge, it must be cleaned and the cycle begun anew.

Tertiary Treatment

As awareness has grown that water is indeed a limited resource, there has been increasing use of treated sewage as a raw water source for industrial processes and as irrigation water for crops and recreational areas (such as golf courses). Such practices conserve water, but the treated effluent must meet certain sanitary standards. In many places the standards are essentially the same as those for drinking water, but researchers continue to try to establish reasonable and cost-effective requirements (World Health Organization, 1989).

Most methods used in tertiary treatment of sewage are modeled on those used in the purification of drinking water: a coagulant is added, a floc is formed and settled, the liquid is then passed through a sand filter, and a disinfectant is added. For certain wastes, however, new and better treatment approaches have been developed specifically to remove organic compounds, heavy metals, and viruses.

For the removal of organic compounds, the usual water treatment process is supplemented by passing the treated waste through two granular carbon beds, each of which provides 30 minutes of contact time. Ozone is applied as a disinfectant to the waste as it passes from the first carbon bed to the second. Heavy metals and viruses are removed by using lime as a coagulant. This process, however, creates large volumes of highly toxic sludge that must be handled and disposed of carefully.

The General Outlook

The provision of water supplies of high quality (almost totally through the use of chlorine as a disinfectant) and in sufficient quantities, and the development of processes for treating and disposing of municipal sewage have promoted an ever-higher level of public health, particularly in the developed countries. In the United States, the National Pollutant Discharge Elimination System has promoted rapid progress in controlling the water environment. The availability of high quality water has also enhanced industrial growth in the United States over the past century. But many problems remain: the presence of an increasing number of toxic chemicals (albeit at low concentrations) such as lead in drinking-water supplies, the production of chlorinated hydrocarbons in the disinfection process, the need to dispose safely of sludges and other wastes produced in the purification of drinking-water supplies and the treatment of municipal sewage and industrial wastes, the rapid depletion of many groundwater supplies, and the contamination of many groundwater supplies with toxic chemicals.

Even efforts to recycle and conserve natural resources have created problems. Attempts to find more uses for the sludge produced in the treatment of municipal sewage must deal with the possibility that the sludge contains many toxic heavy metals. Such materials should not be used as soil builders or as fertilizers lest they enter the food chain.

Another problem is the effectiveness of various sewage treatment processes in removing or destroying pathogenic bacteria and viruses. Conventional primary treatment processes remove only about 50 percent of pathogenic bacteria; and even secondary treatment by the trickling-filter or activated sludge processes removes only about 90 percent. Many viruses also survive these two processes. In the developing countries, the fact that human excreta often mix with drinking-water supplies plays a central role in public health. Fortunately, both double-vault privies and waste stabilization ponds destroy essentially all pathogenic organisms (Mara, 1982).

Recently, the addition of certain polymers to raw sewage has significantly improved primary treatment methods. These "advanced" primary treatment methods significantly increase the amount of solids that settle out and achieve BOD reductions of 75 percent, close to those achieved by secondary treatment systems such as the trickling filter. Furthermore, these methods produce 15–20 percent less sludge than conventional systems using *both* primary and secondary treatment and cost substantially less (Sun, 1989). Some scientists and waste treatment specialists are advocating use of "advanced" primary treatment as a substitute for secondary treatment systems, especially in cities on the seacoast, where sewage treated by this method can be safely discharged into the ocean and serve as a source of food for marine life. Given the increasing U.S. population and the need for improved methods for treating sewage, "advanced" primary treatment may well have a promising future. In any case, as the need for conservation and recycling of water becomes more widely recognized, tertiary treatment of sewage will become common practice.

REFERENCES

Allen, M. J., W. D. Bellamy, J. Bryck, D. W. Hendricks, R. M. Krill, and G. S. Logsdon. 1988. "Slow Sand Filtration." Roundtable discussion. *American Water Works Association Journal* 80, no. 12 (December), 12, 14, 18–19.

Anonymous. 1991. "Vital Signs." *World-Watch* 4, no. 2 (March–April), 6.

Baldwin, Deborah. 1976. "Sludgegate." *Environmental Action* 8, no. 4 (19 June), 3–8.

Canby, Thomas Y. 1980. "Water—Our Most Precious Resource." *National Geographic* 158, no. 2 (August), 144–179.

Chanlett, Emil T. 1979. *Environmental Protection*. 2d ed. New York: McGraw-Hill.

Council on Environmental Quality. 1989. *Environmental Trends*. Washington, D.C.: Executive Office of the President.

Gloyna, Ernest. 1971. *Waste Stabilization Ponds*. Monograph Series no. 60. Geneva: World Health Organization.

Leland, D. E., and M. Damewood III. 1990. "Slow Sand Filtration in Small Systems in Oregon." *American Water Works Association Journal* 82, no. 6 (June), 50–59.

Mara, Duncan. 1982. *Appropriate Technology for Water Supply and Sanitation: Sanitation Alternative for Low-Income Communities—A Brief Introduction*. Washington, D.C.: World Bank.

McKone, Thomas E. 1987. "Human Exposure to Volatile Organic Compounds in Household Tap Water: The Indoor Inhalation Pathway." *Environmental Science & Technology* 21, no. 12 (December), 1194–1201.

Montgomery, James M. 1985. *Water Treatment Principles and Design*. New York: John Wiley and Sons.

National Research Council, Safe Drinking Water Committee. 1977–1989. *Drinking Water and Health*. Vols. 1–9, Washington, D.C.: National Academy Press.

Schroeder, H. A. 1974. "Role of Trace Elements in Cardiovascular Diseases." *Medical Clinics of North America* 58, no. 2, pp. 381–396.

Sun, Marjorie. 1989. "Mud-Slinging over Sewage Technology." *Science* 246, no. 4929 (27 October), 440–443.

UNESCO. 1971. *Scientific Framework of World Water Balance*. Technical Papers in Hydrology, no. 7. Paris.

U.S. Geological Survey. 1988. *Estimated Use of Water in the United States in 1985*. Circular no. 1004. Washington, D.C.

World Health Organization. 1989. *Health Guidelines for Use of Wastewater and Aquaculture*. Technical Report Series no. 778. Geneva.

5

Food

Given the central importance of food in our personal environment, it would appear to be an aspect of our lives over which we have control. Data indicate that this is far from the case. Although the number of reported outbreaks of foodborne disease has shown a decrease in recent years (1983–1987), this success does not apply to all foodborne diseases. A notable example is *Salmonella enteritidis,* which showed a fourfold increase in outbreaks from 1973 to 1987 (Bean and Griffin, 1990). Moreover, outbreaks of foodborne disease are grossly underreported, since many victims do not seek medical care. Only 50,000–100,000 cases of food-related infections are reported each year in the United States, but experts estimate that the actual number of cases is about 5 million (Benenson, 1990).

This chapter focuses on contaminants in food that can be harmful to health. Aside from physical contaminants (such as rust, dirt, hair, machine parts, nails, and bolts), these fall into two broad groups: (1) chemicals, such as lead, cadmium, mercury, sodium, phosphates, nitrites, nitrates, and organic compounds; and (2) biological agents, such as bacteria, viruses, molds, antibiotics, parasites, and their toxins (Figure 5.1). These contaminants can gain access to the food chain at any of a multitude of stages in growing, processing, preparation, and storage.

Chemical Contaminants

Chemical contaminants can occur naturally or may be added during food production or processing.

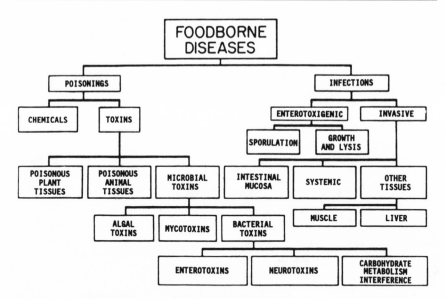

Figure 5.1 Classification of foodborne diseases

Naturally Occurring Contaminants

Many compounds in food plants have been chemically characterized, and a number have been found to be toxic. Although it is generally assumed that the natural components of food, even those known to be toxic, do not constitute an acute health hazard, there is very little information about the toxic effects from ingestion of these compounds over long periods. That certain foods have been consumed for centuries without obvious adverse effects is not sufficient proof in itself that they are safe.

Abnormal and toxic metabolites are frequently produced when plants are subjected to stress. These include protease inhibitors (which are found in many legumes and can inhibit the proteolytic activity of certain enzymes), hemagglutinins (which are found in castor beans, soybeans, black beans, and yellow wax beans and can agglutinate red blood cells), goitrogens (which are found in cabbage, turnips, rutabagas, mustard greens, horseradish, and white mustard and can cause hypothyroidism), and allergens (which are present in peanuts, certain fruits, and grains and cause allergies of the skin and respiratory and gastrointestinal tracts). Certain plants, such as the bracken fern, are poisonous to animals, and the toxins may be present in milk from cows that have eaten the plants.

Chemicals Introduced by Human Activities

Nitrates and Nitrites

Nitrates and nitrites are common ingredients of nitrogen fertilizers and thus can be taken up by vegetables. The concentrations in vegetables vary widely, depending primarily on the species, the concentration of nitrate and molybdenum in the soil, light intensity, and drought conditions. High concentrations of nitrate in baby food, much of which is converted into nitrites, is a cause of methemoglobinemia in infants. Nitrite modifies hemoglobin compounds in the blood so that they cannot transport oxygen from the lungs to the tissues. Methemoglobinemia can be detected in the blood of infants consuming formulas made from water containing high nitrate concentrations. The recommended limit for the nitrate ion in drinking water is 45 milligrams (mg) per liter, which corresponds to about 10 parts per million (ppm) of nitrate-nitrogen. A concentration of about 2 mg of nitrate ion per kilogram of body weight will produce methemoglobinemia in infants.

Sodium Chloride and Phosphate

Sodium is the seventh most plentiful element in the crust of the earth. In its ionized form, sodium enters the food chain either during processing or domestic cooking or at the table. Numerous studies of the effects of sodium chloride intake on human health have yielded contradictory and confusing results, but data do indicate that excessive salt intake is related to hypertension and to gastric injury in some individuals. The estimated average current daily intake of sodium chloride by adults in the United States is 6.8 grams, approximately double the recommended daily intake of 3–4 grams. The recommended daily intake for children and adolescents is 2–3 grams.

Phosphate is being increasingly used in poultry processing and in the production of soft drinks and modified starches. An excessive daily intake of phosphate can lead to premature cessation of bone growth in children and may contribute to osteoporosis in the elderly.

How the human body processes phosphate is influenced by its intake of other chemicals, such as calcium. Good health depends on maintaining a proper ratio in the intake of these two chemicals. The recommended daily intake for adults is about 1,200 mg of phosphate and 1,200–1,800 mg of calcium; that is, the ratio of calcium to phosphate should be about 1.5:1. The recommended daily intake of phosphate for infants is 150 mg.

Metals and Metalloids

Metals such as mercury, lead, and cadmium can have severe effects on human health. Mercury discharged into rivers, lakes, and oceans in the form of inorganic salt or as the metallic element, which is not harmful to humans, can be converted by microbes to alkyl mercury, primarily methyl mercury. In this form mercury can be a significant health hazard. Large-scale poisonings by such compounds have caused deaths and cases of permanent damage to the central nervous system. In a classic episode in Japan in the early 1950s, industrial wastes containing mercury were discharged into Minamata Bay. More than 100 people who ate contaminated fish were poisoned, and 46 died. In the early 1970s tuna and swordfish were recalled from stores in the United States because of mercury concentrations in excess of 0.5 ppm, the limit set by the Food and Drug Administration (FDA). In 1969 a family in New Mexico was severely poisoned after eating pork that contained a methyl mercury fungicide. Similarly, in Iraq in the 1950s people in many parts of the world were poisoned as a result of using cooking oil made from seeds that had been treated with fungicides containing mercury.

The hazards of lead have been known for centuries. Its most salient adverse effects are on the nervous system, the hematopoetic system, and the kidneys. Lead can be ingested indirectly in the form of lead-based paint, drinking water contaminated by the lead pipes that distribute it, metal vessels, pottery glazes, and fungicides that enter the food chain. Before the use of lead was banned from gasoline in the United States, vegetables and other crops from farms located near major roadways were often contaminated with lead through atmospheric deposition. Shellfish may also concentrate lead from contaminated water.

Cadmium has effects similar to those of lead and moves through the environment and into the food chain by similar pathways. A major source of environmental contamination with cadmium comes from discarded batteries such as those used in pocket calculators, cameras, radios, and flashlights. Cadmium affects the kidneys and may be related to hypertension and renal cancer.

Organic Contaminants

Organic contaminants in food include the chlorinated hydrocarbons, polychlorinated biphenyls, chlorinated dibenzo-p-dioxins, and chlorinated dibenzofurans. Their presence in the environment and subsequently in food stems primarily from the use of pesticides and herbicides and the use of polychlorinated biphenyls in heat exchangers in electrical transformers, which sometimes leak or explode. Organic compounds can produce pathological changes in the body, including the stimulation of certain metabolizing enzymes. Such stimulation may have important implications for human health, particularly if the affected enzymes activate or deactivate certain environmental chemicals. Currently, however, very little is known about the mechanisms or significance of these responses.

Antibiotics and Growth Hormones

Today nearly half of all antibiotics produced in the United States are fed to farm animals to prevent disease and to promote growth. Most are broad-spectrum antibiotics such as penicillin or tetracycline (Wright, 1990). This practice is controversial enough that the European Economic Community has threatened to ban the importation of beef from the United States. The transmission of antibiotics through milk and dairy products could affect people who have adverse reactions to certain drugs and, of course, infants and small children. Such practices may also lead to the development of microorganisms that are more resistant to antibiotics. For example, studies have shown that resistance is increasing in *Salmonella* strains (Cohen and Tauxe, 1986). This resistance can lead in turn to the ineffectiveness of antibiotics currently used in medical treatment and the need for newer, often costlier, antibiotics. Although study of possible detrimental effects of the use of antibiotics in animal feed is continuing, no action has been taken to ban it in the United States. As a minimum, however, some experts have called for restricting use to narrow-spectrum anti-biotics that will not result in the development of resistant strains (Wright, 1990).

Similar concerns have been raised over the administration of growth hormones to dairy cows in the United States. The only known effect of growth hormones is an increase in milk production, and the milk contains no undesirable or artificial compounds. However, the European Economic Community has also expressed concern about this practice and has considered banning the importation of milk and other dairy products from countries where cows are receiving such hormones.

Foodborne Illnesses

Table 5.1 summarizes the major foodborne illnesses, including their causes, the food usually involved, and the incubation period. These illnesses may be caused by foodborne parasites, bacterial infections, viral infections, or toxins that either occur naturally in food or are produced by bacteria or viruses.

Foodborne Parasites

Typical parasitic foodborne illnesses include trichinellosis (caused by *Trichinella spiralis*) and giardiasis (caused by *Giardia lamblia*).

Trichinella spiralis (Trichinellosis)

Trichinellosis usually results from the consumption of inadequately cooked pork infested with *Trichinella spiralis,* a nematode or worm. It can also be contracted through beef or horsemeat or through cross-contamination of food. This serious and painful illness shows itself in abdominal pain, vomiting, and malaise at the beginning, and in muscular pain, fever, and fatigue over a longer period. The severity of the illness appears to be related to the number of larvae ingested. Because the symptoms are similar, trichinellosis is often confused with food infections and other diseases. Because it is not possible to detect infected pork at the time of meat inspection, feeding must be carefully monitored. Pigs should be fed only grain, or garbage that has been

Table 5.1 Major foodborne illnesses

Illness	Causative agent	Foods usually involved	Incubation period
Foodborne parasites			
Trichinellosis	*Trichinella spiralis*	Pork	8–15 days
Giardiasis	*Giardiasis lamblia*	Raw salads and vegetables	7–10 days
Amebiasis (amebic dysentery)	*Entamoeba histo-lytica*	Food contaminated with fecal matter	2–4 weeks
Bacterial infections			
Typhoid and para-typhoid fever	*Salmonella typhosa* and *paratyphi A*	Eggs, chicken, pork, beef	12–36 hours
Shigellosis (bacillic dysentery)	*Shigella*	Moist food, milk, dairy products	1–3 weeks
Streptococcal sore throat and scarlet fever	*Beta-hemolytic streptococcus*	Milk products, egg salads	1–3 days
Viral infections			
Viral hepatitis	Hepatitis A	Sandwiches, salads	28–30 days
Foodborne toxins			
Paralytic shellfish poisoning	Dinoflagellates (neurotoxins)	Shellfish	Up to 24 hours
Cancer	*Aspergillus flavus* (mycotoxins)	Peanuts, corn, cereal grains	Years
Staphylococcal food poisoning	*Staphylococcus aureus*	Meat, poultry, custards, salad dressings, sandwiches	2–4 hours
Botulism	*Clostridium botu-linum*	Home-canned vegetables, fruit	12–36 hours
Gastroenteritis	*Clostridium per-fringens*	Meat, poultry, vegetables, spices	10–12 hours
Diarrhea	*Escherichia coli*	Meat, poultry, shellfish, watercress	24–72 hours

thoroughly cooked. In any case, all pork products intended for human consumption should be thoroughly cooked.

Giardia lamblia (Giardiasis)

Giardiasis is a protozoan infection principally of the upper small intestine. *Giardia* cysts are present in human stools worldwide, ranging in prevalence from 1 percent to 30 percent depending on the community and age group surveyed. Children are infected more frequently than adults. The asymptomatic carrier rate is high. The disease shows itself in diarrhea, fever, or both and in flatulence, nausea, malaise, or abdominal cramps. Often the organism enters the body through the consumption of contaminated water or through person-to-person transmission. Localized outbreaks may also occur from ingestion of food that has been fecally contaminated by handlers. Foodborne outbreaks are on the increase, one source being the "open" salad bars that have become common in many restaurants. Specific sources that have been identified include home-prepared salmon and fruit salads contaminated by *Giardia* cysts (Porter et al., 1990).

Bacterial Infections

Certain bacteria can gain access to foods and be ingested and transported to the digestive tract, where they can multiply and cause illnesses. Common examples are *Salmonella, Streptococci,* and *Shigella.*

Salmonella (Salmonellosis)

Salmonella exist in the intestines of chickens, dogs, and rodents. These bacteria can also live in the ambient environment and can survive conditions that many other organisms cannot. This resistance accounts for their transmission through drinking water as well as food. Once ingested, *Salmonella* multiply in the intestines and cause fever and diarrhea within 12–36 hours.

In 1986 37 percent of the chicken, 12 percent of the pork, and 5 percent of the beef inspected by the U.S. Department of Agriculture was contaminated with *Salmonella* (Rubel, 1987). Eggs and poultry are primary sources of infection. Formerly, transmission of *Salmo-*

nella through eggs was thought to involve contamination on the outside of the shell. Today, however, the organisms are often present inside eggs, as a result of infections in the ovaries of chickens. All protein foods requiring a large amount of handling are subject to contamination. Low-acid foods, such as meat pies, custard-filled bakery products, and improperly cooked sausages, are common sources of *Salmonella* outbreaks. Transmission can be prevented by pasteurization of frozen eggs and thorough cooking.

Shigella (Shigellosis—Bacillic Dysentery)

Bacillic dysentery is caused by *Shigella dysenteriae,* an infectious agent common wherever sanitation is a problem. Two-thirds of all cases, and most deaths, occur in children under 10 years of age. Illness in infants less than 6 months old is unusual. Secondary attack rates in households can be as high as 40 percent. *Shigella* are commonly present in human feces, and transmission is favored by crowded conditions, where personal contact is unavoidable. Food handlers can readily spread the infection through contamination of food. Flies can also transfer the organisms to nonrefrigerated food, where they can multiply. Ingestion of a relatively large number of organisms is required, and onset of the disease is delayed for 1–3 weeks, while the bacteria multiply in the body. Personal cleanliness, particularly in handling food, is an important factor in the control of this disease (Benenson, 1990).

Beta-Hemolytic Streptococcus (Streptococcal Sore Throat and Scarlet Fever)

Beta-hemolytic streptococcus causes streptococcal sore throat and scarlet fever. Streptococcal sore throat patients frequently exhibit fever, sore throat, tonsillitis, and tender lymph nodes. Scarlet fever is characterized by a skin rash. Streptococcal sore throat and scarlet fever are common in temperate zones, well recognized and diagnosed in semitropical areas, and less frequently recognized in tropical climates. Explosive outbreaks of streptococcal sore throat may follow ingestion of contaminated food. Milk and milk products have been associated most frequently with foodborne outbreaks; egg salad and deviled hard-boiled eggs have recently been implicated with increasing frequency (Benenson, 1990). Although scarlet fever is more often transmitted by direct person-to-person contact, transmission has also been traced to the consumption of raw milk, which is also a principal carrier in cases of streptococcal sore throat. To prevent the growth of the organism, milk should be held at a temperature of 50°F (10°C). Milk products and protein mixtures such as egg salad may also carry the organism if they are not made from pasteurized products.

Viral Infections

Infectious hepatitis (Hepatitis A) is a highly contagious disease caused by a virus whose symptoms are fever and general discomfort. This disease occurs most frequently among school-age children and young adults. The infectious agent is commonly present in feces. Common-source outbreaks have been related to food, such as sandwiches and salads, that is not cooked or is handled after cooking by infected foodhandlers. Raw or undercooked mollusks harvested from contaminated waters may also be sources of infection. In the United States an estimated 1,000 cases each year are attributed to suspected food- or waterborne sources. An outbreak in 1988 was traced to commercially distributed lettuce. Certain commercially processed food, such as frozen raspberries, appears to be associated with transmission of the virus in the United Kingdom (Rosenblum et al., 1990).

Foodborne Toxins

Foodborne illnesses may also be caused by the ingestion of toxins naturally present in plants or animals, or subsequently produced in food as a result of contamination by bacteria, viruses, and fungi.

Naturally Occurring Toxins

Of the many toxins that occur naturally in plants and animals, several have been specifically associated with human illness. The most dramatic example is paralytic shellfish poisoning, caused by a highly poisonous neurotoxin (Red Tide) that is a metabolite of certain marine dinoflagellates. Ingestion of shellfish that have fed on this metabolite can quickly lead to death. Toxins can also be produced in plants by naturally occurring fungi. Since many toxigenic fungi can thrive in a wide variety of environmental situations, it is not surprising that there are numerous recorded episodes of human and livestock illnesses and deaths resulting from the ingestion of food or feed contaminated with fungal toxins.

The term *mycotoxin* refers to any toxic fungal metabolite; diseases resulting from exposure to mycotoxins are called *mycotoxicoses*. The best-characterized mycotoxicoses are those in which mycotoxins were consumed in amounts high enough to result in immediate signs of illness or death. In most of these cases, the level of fungal invasion of the responsible food or feed was substantial, and mold damage was highly visible. Humans consumed the infected food either because they were ignorant of the possible consequences or because no other food was available. Mycotoxicoses have been far more common in animals than in humans simply because livestock are more likely to be fed mold-damaged feed.

The discovery in the 1960s of a specific group of mycotoxins known as the aflatoxins added new dimensions to this problem. Mycotoxicoses can no longer be considered as occurring only as a result of severe mold invasion of food, as limited mainly to agriculturally primitive regions, and as preventable simply by handling and storing agricultural commodities in ways that avert serious mold growth. Experience has shown that aflatoxins can readily contaminate certain primary food and feed, such as peanuts, corn, and other cereal grains, and tree nuts. Studies are needed to determine whether contamination takes place in the field or during harvest, transport, and storage. Some aflatoxins have immediately acute effects. Others take their toll through chronic exposure; in one case the result is primary liver cancer (Nelson and Whittenberger, 1977).

Toxins from Improper Food Handling

In contrast to the bacterial infections described above, which are caused directly by the organisms themselves, some foodborne illnesses are caused by the toxins produced by bacteria that are not in themselves harmful. Four principal types of bacteria produce harmful toxins.

STAPHYLOCOCCUS AUREUS (STAPHYLOCOCCAL FOOD POISONING)

If present in food under the proper conditions, *Staphylococcus aureus* will produce one or more enterotoxins that can lead to foodborne illness. In fact this organism is one of the principal sources of acute foodborne illnesses in the United States. Ingestion of contaminated food causes acute intestinal disturbance, usually within 2–4 hours. *Staphylococcus aureus* can readily be transmitted to food from infected cuts, boils, sores, postnasal drip, or sprays expelled during coughing or sneezing. Meat (especially ham), meat products, poultry, poultry products, and poultry dressing are common offenders. Custards used for pastry fillings have likewise been involved in outbreaks of food poisoning. The enterotoxins have also been found to develop in inadequately cured hams and salami and in nonprocessed and inadequately processed cheese. *Staphylococci* are present in air, water, milk, and sewage, and they grow rapidly, especially in food held at room temperature for several hours before being eaten. Refrigeration after cooking provides effective control.

CLOSTRIDIUM BOTULISM (BOTULISM)

Botulism is caused by the ingestion of food containing the toxins produced by *Clostridium botulinum*. This organism will grow in food, particularly under conditions of reduced oxygen. The spores of the bacillus may be present in all types of food, especially spoiled vegetable or animal matter. Underprocessed food and preserved food provide ideal environments. The toxins can exist for long periods, are very resistant to destruction by heat, and are very potent; a small quantity can cause death. In fact these toxins are generally considered to be the most potent produced by any biological organism.

Five types of *Clostridia* have been identified as causing botulism, each varying in the degree of toxicity to its host: Type A, the most common cause of botulism, including infant botulism, found in most soils and in home-canned vegetables; Type B, found in most soils but less toxic than Type A; Type C, a common cause of botulism in poultry, cattle, and horses; Type D, a common cause of botulism in cattle; and Type E, which is toxic to humans and commonly originates through the ingestion of fish and fish products. Specific antitoxins are available for each type of botulism. Heating food to 212°F (100°C) will destroy the organisms; destruction of the spores, however, requires prolonged heating. Swelling or bulging canned goods do not necessarily indicate the presence of spore-forming bacteria, but goods in such containers should not be consumed.

CLOSTRIDIUM PERFRINGENS (GASTROENTERITIS)

Clostridium perfringens gastroenteritis is a mild illness, and those afflicted seldom seek medical treatment. As a result, its frequency of occurrence is undoubtedly underreported. *Clostridium perfringens* is widely distributed and can usually be found in soil, dust, human feces, and animal manure. Meat and poultry are frequently contaminated, as are vegetables and spices. Although *Clostridium* rarely produces spores while growing in food, it does produce spores in the intestinal tract. The spores are very resistant to heat; some can withstand boiling temperatures for up to 6 hours, so even cooked food is frequently contaminated. Once in the human intestine, the organism multiplies and produces an enterotoxin, which in turn produces diarrhea and abdominal cramps. The illness is self-limiting, so treatment is supportive not curative. Prevention requires inhibiting germination of the spores and proliferation of the vegetative cells. This can be accomplished by holding cooked food at a temperature either high enough (above 133°F; 56°C) or low enough (below 64°F; 18°C) that *Clostridium perfringens* cannot multiply (Bryan, 1980).

ESCHERICHIA COLI (GASTROENTERITIS)

Escherichia coli, one of the common causes of traveler's diarrhea, are present in the lower intestinal tract of most warm-blooded animals and are the most prevalent oxygen-tolerant bacteria in the large intestine of humans. They are transferred from feces and intestinal contents to carcasses and meat during processing. Shellfish and watercress can be contaminated if grown in sewage-contaminated waters. The enterotoxigenic strains cause illness within 8–44 hours after infection. Diarrhea usually ceases within 30 hours. Contamination with *Escherichia coli* can be minimized or prevented by good personal hygiene during food handling. Outbreaks can be prevented by heating food long enough and at temperatures high enough to destroy the bacteria, and then cooling the food at temperatures sufficiently low (below 40°F; 4°C) to prevent their proliferation. Also essential are a safe drinking-water supply and proper methods of sewage disposal (Bryan, 1980).

Food Preservation

There is a variety of safe methods for preserving wholesome food, preventing contamination, and destroying organisms or toxins that may have gained access to or been produced within it. Effective use of these methods requires an understanding of the factors that affect bacterial growth.

> *Acidity and alkalinity:* Most bacteria grow best in a neutral medium; highly acid or alkaline media inhibit growth. Most bacteria that contaminate food require oxygen for growth.
>
> *Moisture:* Most bacteria will grow on moist surfaces or in water. Each kind has an upper and a lower limit of growth activity in solution, depending on whether salt, sugars, or other materials are present.
>
> *Temperature:* Each kind of bacteria has maximum, optimum, and minimum temperatures at which growth proceeds. Most disease organisms grow best at the normal temperature of the human body (98.6°F; 37°C). Temperatures above 160°F (71°C) will kill most organisms; temperatures below 40°F (5°C) will retard their growth.

Most bacteria, then, will grow rapidly under warm and moist conditions, contaminating any food in which they are present. However, certain bacteria are very useful, particularly in the fermentation of food; examples include bread, yogurt, and wine. In these cases, their growth and the changes they produce are essential to their beneficial effects.

Cooking

Cooking renders food digestible and palatable. Although it also tends to kill many bacteria, this process alone will not preserve food. In fact cooking may render protein foods (meat, eggs, milk, and milk products) more susceptible to bacterial growth, permitting active increases in the number of harmful organisms or the toxins they may produce. Unless food is heated thoroughly and to a high enough temperature, any microorganisms present will not be killed. Even if they are killed, the cooked food must be eaten promptly or protected from subsequent spoilage.

Canning

The process of canning consists in heating food to a sufficient degree to kill any microorganisms present and then sealing it in a container to keep it sterile. The combination of time and temperature required to preserve food by canning varies with the product and its likely contaminants. Acid foods, such as tomatoes and some fruits, need to be heated to the boiling point for only a few minutes. Nonacid foods, such as corn and beans, must be heated to higher temperatures (under pressure) for a longer time to prevent undesirable changes in appearance and flavor.

Drying and Dehydration

Air drying is one of the most economical and effective ways of preserving food and has been practiced for centuries. Today food can be dried in the sun or by artificial heating processes. Other methods of drying include spray drying, freeze drying, vacuum drying, and hot-air drying. However, once the food is reconstituted by the addition of water, bacterial activity resumes, and sanitary control is essential.

Preservatives

Certain preservatives can be used to inhibit the growth of microorganisms or to kill them. Salt, sugar, sodium nitrate, and nitrites are commonly used for curing and pickling meats and vegetables; often other agents such as salicylic acid and sodium benzoate are added too. Ordinarily, meats can be preserved by a combination of salting, curing, and smoking. Corned beef, however, must subsequently be refrigerated. Smoking often improves flavor and helps inhibit microbial growth. Propionates and sorbic acid are commonly used to prevent mold formation in breads.

Refrigeration

Storing food at temperatures lower than 40°F (5°C) will retard the growth of pathogenic organisms and the more important spoilage organisms, but it does not prevent all changes. The level of humidity is also important: too little results in moisture loss; too much promotes the growth of spoilage organisms. Proper air circulation and regular cleaning and sanitizing of chill spaces are mandatory.

Freezing

Although bacteria that cause food spoilage do not multiply at freezing temperatures, once thawing begins frozen food becomes vulnerable to bacteria and the associated toxins they may produce. As a result, refreezing will not make the food safe. Nor will freezing improve the original quality of the product. Thus, the selection of good products for freezing is essential. One variation of freezing is "dehydrofreezing," in which the food is partially dehydrated (but still perishable) and then frozen. This process provides the space and weight savings of dehydration without depriving food of its fresh color, flavor, and palatability.

Pasteurization

Pasteurization is an excellent method for preserving food for a short time. Combined with refrigeration, it extends the useful shelf life of dairy products. Milk is generally heated to 145°F (63°C) for 30 minutes—or to 161°F (72°C) for 15 seconds—to kill the pathogenic organisms. Although some heat-resistant organisms will survive, subsequent refrigeration will preserve the milk for up to several weeks.

Irradiation

The use of ionizing radiation to preserve food has been proposed for many years but has not been widely accepted or applied. The process consists in subjecting food to ionizing radiation at sufficiently high doses to kill a large fraction of any microorganisms it contains. No radioactive material (frequently the source of the radiation) is permitted to come into contact with the food, and the final product is not radioactive. However, in some food the process does produce unwanted changes in taste and palatability, and fears persist that irradiation may produce new chemical products in the food that could be carcinogenic. The FDA has approved irradiation as a means of controlling foodborne pathogens in poultry, inhibiting sprouting in white potatoes, and preserving spices. The process is being used in commercial food processing in Canada, Japan, and the USSR. Because of public opposition, however, spices are the only food product routinely being treated with radiation in the United States (Food and Drug Administration, 1990).

Sanitation in Food Handling

Prevention and control of foodborne illnesses require an effective sanitation program. Data on the nature and sources of the major problems involved are essential components of such a program. Table 5.2 summarizes the contributions of a range of food preparation and handling operations to outbreaks of various types of foodborne illnesses in the United States for the years 1973–1987. Table 5.3 summarizes the relative contributions of these operations to reported outbreaks of foodborne illness involving specific types of food products for the same period.

Also essential to a sound food sanitation program are a safe water supply, adequate garbage and refuse disposal, proper wastewater and sewage disposal, and effective insect and rodent control (Chapters 4 and 7). Other factors include equipment and facilities, personnel, standards, and inspection.

Equipment and Facilities

Equipment used in the preparation or processing of food should be designed to facilitate cleaning. Vehicles used to transport food products must be clean and should not be used to transport any other products. Refrigerated vehicles must be available for the transport of perishable food.

Facilities should be designed so that all food, particularly vegetables, can be stored above the floor where they will remain dry and will not come into contact with powders and sprays applied to control insects and rodents.

Personnel: Training and Habits

In the handling and preparation of food products, personal hygiene is indispensable. Food handlers must (1) wash their hands after toilet use and before and after work; (2) avoid contact between open wounds and foodstuffs; (3) wear clean outer garments, including a cap over the hair; and (4) avoid using tobacco products while working. The use of tobacco can lead to contamination of the fingers and hands with saliva and may promote spitting, which can transfer disease organisms to the food or to surfaces with which it comes into contact. Food handlers should also be trained in appropriate methods of food storage, garbage disposal, and insect and rodent control.

Standards and Inspection

Laws that stipulate procedures for growing, processing, storing, handling, and distributing food products must be based on appropriate standards, and funding must be sufficient to assure adequate inspection and enforcement, supported by the various laboratory tests necessary for determining whether food samples are wholesome.

The General Outlook

For most of the many illnesses that can be transmitted to humans through the consumption of food, both the mechanisms by which they operate and the steps necessary for their control are known. The control of foodborne illnesses extends beyond immediate production and processing. A safe food supply requires water supplies of adequate quality and quantity, proper methods for disposing of human excreta, education of food handlers in safe and sanitary procedures, and, indeed, public education. All individuals must assume some responsibility for assuring that their food is as clean as reasonably possible, that their overall diet is balanced in nutrients, and that they handle and store food safely. Table 5.4 lists the essential rules for safe food preparation.

In many parts of the world, an inadequate food supply is the foremost problem. Recent droughts have led to reduced food production and to famine in many localities. Today the quantity and quality of the food supply are being addressed together. Through selection and breeding, plants are being developed that grow more rapidly, produce higher yields, or can be irrigated with salt water (National Research Council, 1990). Through advances in molecular biology and biotechnology, plants are being made more resistant to pathogens, more uni-

Table 5.2 Contributing factors to foodborne illnesses caused by specific etiologic agent, 1973–1987

Etiologic agent	Number of outbreaks in which factors were reported[b]	Contributing factor[a]					
		Improper storage or holding temperature	Inadequate cooking	Contaminated equipment	Food from unsafe source	Poor personal hygiene	Other
Bacterial							
Bacillus cereus	48	94	32	53	5	24	33
Brucella	2	0	50	0	100	0	100
Campylobacter	27	45	45	45	67	45	57
Clostridium botulinum	69	34	91	3	3	0	41
Clostridium perfringens	147	97	65	28	6	26	34
Escherichia coli	3	—	50	0	0	0	100
Salmonella	504	83	67	63	25	63	43
Shigella	68	63	3	30	11	91	33
Staphylococcus aureus	272	98	22	43	12	71	24
Streptococcus, group A	11	100	0	0	0	88	20
Streptococcus, other	2	—	—	—	100	100	0
Vibrio cholerae	3	100	100	—	100	—	—
Vibrio cholerae, non-01	1	—	100	—	100	—	—
Vibrio parahaemolyticus	16	75	92	0	75	0	33
Yersinia enterocolitica	2	100	100	100	100	100	100
Other bacterial	7	100	50	0	50	100	100
Total	1,182	87	56	47	20	59	37

Viral							
Hepatitis A	55	21	21	19	19	96	21
Norwalk virus	11	50	33	50	60	78	50
Other virus	5	67	67	50	0	80	67
Total	71	28	26	26	23	92	29
Parasitic							
Giardia	2	0	0	0	0	100	0
Trichinella spiralis	74	13	100	7	24	0	4
Other parasitic	4	0	100	0	0	0	0
Total	80	12	99	6	22	6	3
Chemical							
Ciguatoxin	68	9	0	0	82	0	74
Heavy metals	39	25	0	58	20	7	78
Monosodium glutamine	8	0	0	0	0	0	88
Mushroom poisoning	43	0	0	0	98	0	6
Paralytic shellfish poisoning	14	0	0	0	100	0	50
Histamine (scombroid) fish poisoning	102	83	0	8	52	3	48
Other chemical	71	11	6	23	34	3	85
Total	345	42	2	17	66	2	67

a. Percentage of outbreaks in which this factor was a contributor.
b. Number of outbreaks for which the presence or absence of any factor was reported. The denominator for each factor varies and is the number of outbreaks in which the presence or absence of that factor was reported.

Table 5.3   Contributing factors to illnesses transmitted through various food products, 1973–1987

Food product	Number of outbreaks in which factors were reported[b]	Contributing factor[a]					
		Improper storage or holding temperature	Inadequate cooking	Contaminated equipment	Food from unsafe source	Poor personal hygiene	Other
Bakery products	51	73	12	57	22	67	35
Beef	209	94	61	50	12	55	39
Chicken	80	89	70	45	4	47	29
Chinese food	90	91	23	58	0	51	62
Dairy products	60	32	32	17	82	18	63
Eggs	25	88	43	25	14	59	25
Finfish	228	68	27	13	58	19	49
Fruits, vegetables	67	40	55	25	17	29	46
Ice cream	30	47	84	27	65	21	47
Mexican food	93	92	42	33	4	32	26
Mushrooms	47	0	10	0	93	0	11
Nondairy beverages	65	32	10	41	25	13	72
Pork	170	90	50	43	14	53	17
Shellfish	145	60	75	13	87	29	30
Turkey	91	95	68	45	14	50	30
Other	775	82	43	40	12	55	41

a. Percentage of outbreaks to which this factor was a contributor.
b. Number of outbreaks for which the presence or absence of any factor was reported. The denominator for each factor varies and is the number of outbreaks in which the presence or absence of that factor was reported.

Table 5.4   10 rules for safe food preparation

 1. Choose food processed for safety.
 2. Cook food thoroughly.
 3. Eat cooked food immediately.
 4. Store cooked food immediately.
 5. Reheat cooked foods thoroughly.
 6. Avoid contact between raw and cooked foods.
 7. Wash hands repeatedly.
 8. Keep all kitchen surfaces meticulously clean.
 9. Protect foods from insects, rodents and other animals.
10. Use pure water.

form in composition, higher in quality, and higher in concentrations of desirable compounds, such as beta carotene.

One adverse result of attempts to increase crop yields is greater use of chemical fertilizers, with higher runoffs that threaten more pollution of lakes and rivers. This result highlights the need for a systems approach in developing methods to assure a safe and adequate food supply. Only if environmental and public health officials are armed with a full understanding of the multitude of factors involved will they be able to minimize potential risks both to the public and to the environment.

REFERENCES

Bean, N. H., and P. M. Griffin. 1990. "Foodborne Disease Outbreaks in the United States, 1973–1987: Pathogens, Vehicles, and Trends." *Journal of Food Protection* 53, no. 9 (September), 804–817.

Benenson, Abram S., ed. 1990. *Control of Communicable Diseases in Man.* 15th ed. Washington, D.C.: American Public Health Association.

Bryan, F. L. 1980. *Foodborne Diseases and Their Control.* Atlanta: Centers for Disease Control, U.S. Department of Health and Human Services.

Cohen, Mitchell L., and Robert V. Tauxe. 1986. "Drug-Resistant *Salmonella* in the United States: An Epidemiologic Perspective." *Science* 234 (21 November), 964–969.

Food and Drug Administration, U.S. Department of Health and Human Services. 1990. "21 CFR Part 179, Irradiation in the Production, Processing, and Handling of Food: Final Rule." *Federal Register,* 2 May, pp. 18538–44.

National Research Council. 1990. "The Growing Promise of Salt-Tolerant Plants." *NewsReport* 40, no. 5 (May), 2–4.

Nelson, Norton, and James W. Whittenberger. 1977. *Human Health and the Environment: Some Research Needs*. DHEW Publication NIH 77-1277. Washington, D.C.: U.S. Government Printing Office.

Porter, J. D. H., C. Gaffney, D. Heymann, and W. Parkin. 1990. "Foodborne Outbreak of Giardia Lamblia." *American Journal of Public Health* 80, no. 10 (October), 1259–60.

Rosenblum, L. S., I. R. Mirkin, D. T. Allen, S. Safford, and S. C. Hadler. 1990. "A Multifocal Outbreak of Hepatitis A Traced to Commercially Distributed Lettuce." *American Journal of Public Health* 80, no. 9 (September), 1075–80.

Rubel, Judith, ed. 1987. *To Your Health!* Lahey Clinic Health Letter. Burlington, Mass.

Wright, Karen. 1990. "The Policy Response: In Limbo" [on the use of antibiotics in animal feeds]. *Science* 249, no. 4964 (6 July), 24.

6

Solid Waste

Until World War II, most solid or municipal waste took the form of garbage, yard waste (including leaves, grass clippings, and tree limbs), newspapers, cans and bottles, coal and wood ashes, street sweepings, and discarded building materials. Most such waste was not considered hazardous, and it was simply transported to the town land disposal facility or "dump," where it was periodically set on fire to reduce its volume and to discourage the breeding of insects and rodents. Because this practice often led to windblown debris and generally unsightly disposal facilities, and because people recognized the need for a technically sounder method of disposal, this approach was gradually replaced by the sanitary landfill where municipal waste is buried in the ground (Figure 6.1). As long as windblown debris and fires were contained, material was covered over and sealed daily (so that breeding and habitation by insects and rodents were controlled), and contamination of nearby groundwater supplies was avoided, sanitary landfills were considered an acceptable method of disposal.

Since World War II, with the development of a "throwaway" society and an unprecedented demand for new products, the volume of solid waste has enormously increased and its composition has changed. Solid waste today contains many materials, such as plastics, that are not readily degradable, and toxic materials—primarily various types of chemical waste produced by industry—that can contaminate soil and groundwater indefinitely if not properly disposed of. Developing methods for the management and disposal of such waste has been a formidable challenge.

The United States produces more municipal solid waste and hazardous waste per capita than any other industrialized nation (Council, 1989). On the average each person in the United States produces

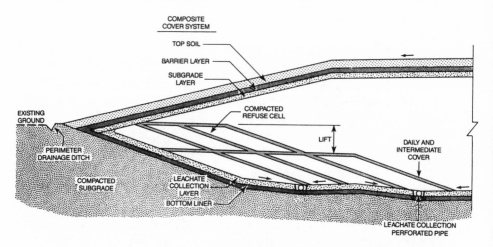

Figure 6.1   Cross-section of a typical landfill and leachate collection system

1,000–1,500 pounds of municipal solid waste, including almost 100 pounds of plastics, per year. In addition, industry produces the equivalent of over one ton of hazardous waste per person each year. In 1987 industry discharged 18 billion pounds of toxic chemicals directly into the air, water, or land or into deep underground injection wells, and another 4.6 billion pounds were transferred off-site to other facilities, such as public sewage systems or incinerators, for treatment and disposal (EPA, 1989). Also requiring management are the vast quantities of sludges produced in the purification of drinking water, the treatment of sewage and industrial waste, the operation of air-cleaning equipment (scrubbers) in power plants, and high- and low-level radioactive wastes produced by the operation of nuclear power plants and the use of radioactive materials in medicine, research, and industry.

About 80 percent of the solid waste produced in the United States goes to sanitary landfills (Langone, 1989). However, establishing new facilities is becoming more and more difficult, and existing disposal sites are being filled and phased out, so the number of landfills in operation has been decreasing. In 1985 there were about 9,000; in 1990 there were 6,000; and 2,000 more are expected to be closed by the end of 1993 (Donahue, 1988).

Federal Regulations

In 1965 Congress first acknowledged the need for action in the management and disposal of solid waste by passing the Solid Waste Disposal Act. This legislation established grant programs to support the use of improved methods for disposal and the development of solid waste disposal plans by states, interstate agencies, or both. In 1976 the Resource Conservation and Recovery Act (RCRA) clarified the definitions of solid waste and responded to growing public concerns about leakage and contamination of groundwater supplies from an estimated 100,000–300,000 underground storage tanks containing hazardous substances or petroleum products (Table 6.1). Subsequent laws have continued to address the management and disposal of solid and hazardous waste (Table 6.2). In fact this has become the most

Table 6.1   Principal programs and goals of the Resource Conservation
and Recovery Act (1976)

Solid Waste Program (directed primarily at management and control of nonhazardous solid wastes)

Primary goals:
To encourage environmentally sound solid-waste management practices
To maximize reuse of recoverable resources
To foster resource conservation

Hazardous Waste Program ("cradle-to-grave" system for managing hazardous waste)

Primary goals:
To identify hazardous waste
To regulate generators and transporters of hazardous waste
To regulate owners and operators of facilities that treat, store, or dispose of hazardous waste

Underground Storage Tank Program

Primary goals:
To provide performance standards for new tanks
To prohibit installation of unprotected new tanks
To provide regulations concerning leak detection, prevention, and corrective action

Table 6.2   Principal federal laws related to management and disposal
of solid and hazardous waste

Year	Law	Public Law number
1965	Solid Waste Disposal Act	89-272
1976	Resource Conservation and Recovery Act (RCRA)	94-580
1980	Comprehensive Environmental Response, Compensation, and Liability Act (Superfund Act)	96-150
1984	Hazardous and Solid Waste Amendments, Resource Conservation and Recovery Act	98-616
1986	Superfund Amendments and Reauthorization Act (SARA)	99-499

heavily regulated and costly area of environmental protection (Linnerooth and Kneese, 1989).

Overall Objectives

Underlying all these laws are the goals of the RCRA:

To protect human health and the environment from the potential
  hazards of waste disposal
To conserve energy and natural resources
To reduce the amount of waste generated
To ensure that wastes are managed in an environmentally sound
  manner

The RCRA is administered by the EPA, which has issued regulations for its implementation under Title 40, Parts 240–271, of the Code of Federal Regulations (EPA, 1986a, 1986b). The regulatory system's "cradle-to-grave" approach features detailed recordkeeping requirements, a complex permit process, strict financial liability for waste generators and transporters, and a cleanup fund drawn from private sources (Figure 6.2). This fund was mandated by the Comprehensive Environmental Response, Compensation, and Liability Act of 1980, commonly called the CERCLA or Superfund Act. The Superfund Act focuses on the cleanup of sites where toxic chemical waste has been improperly discharged or buried. To prevent the creation of more such sites, the 1984 amendments to the Solid Waste Act restrict the disposal of many wastes on land and emphasize source reduction and recycling (Linnerooth and Kneese, 1989).

The RCRA requires active maintenance of hazardous waste disposal facilities for 30 years but no long-term institutional control. Nor is the waste required to be in any specified form (for example, solidified). At best, the law provides for safe intermediate storage of hazardous waste, which may well have to be reclaimed and treated sometime in the future.

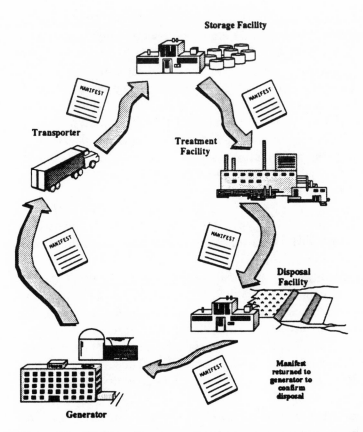

Figure 6.2 The "cradle-to-grave" management system for hazardous waste, from generation to ultimate disposal

Definitions of Solid and Hazardous Waste

Solid waste comes in a variety of types and classes. As a general rule, the waste produced by homeowners is designated as municipal nonhazardous waste, and the toxic chemical waste produced by industry is classified as hazardous. Solid waste is also produced by the treatment of liquid and airborne wastes. For example, chemical treatment of liquid waste produces sludges, and processes for removing pollutants, such as sulfur oxides, from airborne releases produce solid waste. One of the primary objectives of the Resource Conservation and Recovery Act was to clarify the definition of solid waste and to establish a distinction between solid nonhazardous and hazardous waste.

The RCRA defined solid (nonhazardous) waste as "any garbage, refuse, sludge from a waste treatment plant, water supply treatment plant, or air pollution control facility and other discarded material, including solid, liquid, semisolid, or contained gaseous material resulting from industrial, commercial, mining, and agricultural operations and from community activities, but does not include solid or dissolved material in domestic sewage" (EPA, 1986a). Examples of such waste include domestic trash and garbage, such as milk cartons and coffee grounds; other refuse, such as metal scrap, wallboard, and empty containers; and other discarded materials from industrial operations, such as boiler slag and fly ash.

By this definition, solid waste includes hazardous waste, that is, hazardous waste is a subset of solid waste. However, the RCRA treated hazardous waste separately and defined it as including any "solid waste, or combination of solid wastes, which because of its quantity, concentration, or physical, chemical, or infectious characteristics may: (1) cause, or significantly contribute to an increase in mortality or an increase in serious irreversible, or incapacitating illness; or (2) pose a substantial present or potential hazard to human health or the environment when improperly treated, stored, transported, or disposed of, or otherwise managed." Thus, a material cannot be classified as a hazardous waste unless it is first defined as a solid waste.

The EPA has specified that a solid waste is hazardous if analysis proves it to be (1) ignitable, (2) corrosive, (3) reactive, or (4) toxic. Title 40, Parts 261.31–261.33 of the Code of Federal Regulations lists almost 300 substances as hazardous wastes. According to the EPA, the chemical and petroleum industries generate over 70 percent of the hazardous waste in the United States (EPA, 1986a). The rest comes from a wide range of other industries, including metal finishing, general manufacturing, and transportation (Table 6.3).

One subcategory of hazardous waste that has recently aroused concern is medical waste, which contains infectious materials, including needles and plastic syringes. Soon after these wastes were observed washing up on ocean beaches in the summer of 1989, Congress directed the EPA to gather data on their sources, associated health hazards, and current procedures and regulations for management and disposal; and to evaluate the health hazards associated with transporting them, incinerating them, burying them in a landfill, and disposing of them in a sanitary sewer system (EPA, 1990). Table 6.4 summarizes the EPA's initial findings on the sources of medical waste. Not surprisingly, hospitals, long-term health care facilities, and physicians' offices are the major producers of these wastes, which account for about 0.3 percent by weight of all municipal waste. The EPA found that current practices range from handling the waste as nonhazardous municipal solid waste, to strict segregation, packaging, labeling, and tracking from the generator to the disposal site. Common treatment techniques include steam sterilization and incineration.

Under the current regulatory structure, commercially generated waste is classified as nonhazardous, hazardous, mixed, or radioactive. Table 6.5 summarizes the characteristics, volumes, and groups responsible for regulating each category. As the table shows, chemical wastes may be classified as either hazardous or nonhazardous. Similarly, radioactive wastes that do not contain hazardous chemicals are classified as radioactive, and those that contain both radioactive materials and toxic chemicals are classified as mixed.

Management and Disposal of Hazardous Waste

The primary method for managing and disposing of hazardous waste is burial in the ground. Incineration may be used before disposal. Land disposal includes a range of options (EPA, 1986b):

Landfills: Disposal facilities in which hazardous waste is placed in or on land. In most landfills, the wastes are isolated in discrete

Table 6.3 Examples of hazardous waste generated by business and industry

Waste generator	Type of waste
Chemical manufacturers	Strong acids and bases Spent solvents Reactive wastes
Vehicle maintenance shops	Paint wastes containing heavy metals Ignitable wastes Used lead acid batteries Spent solvents
Printing industry	Heavy metal solutions Waste inks Spent solvents Spent electroplating wastes Ink sludges containing heavy metals
Leather products manufacturing	Waste toluene and benzene
Paper industry	Paint wastes containing heavy metals Ignitable solvents Strong acids and bases
Construction industry	Ignitable paint wastes Spent solvents Strong acids and bases
Cleaning agents and cosmetics manufacturing	Heavy metal dusts Ignitable wastes Flammable solvents Strong acids and bases
Furniture and wood manufacturing and refinishing	Ignitable wastes Spent solvents
Metal manufacturing	Paint wastes containing heavy metals Strong acids and bases Cyanide wastes Sludges containing heavy metals

cells within trenches. Properly designed and operated landfills must have double liners to prevent leakage, systems to collect any leachate (should the liners fail) and any surface water runoff that may become contaminated, and wells for periodic sampling to assure that the liners are not leaking (Figure 6.3).

Surface impoundments: Natural or man-made depressions or diked areas that can be used to treat, store, or dispose of hazardous waste. Surface impoundments may be of any shape or size (ranging from a few hundred square feet to hundreds of acres). Surface impoundments are often called pits, ponds, lagoons, and basins.

Underground injection wells: Steel- and concrete-encased shafts placed deep in the earth into which wastes are injected under pressure. Liquid hazardous wastes are commonly disposed of in this manner.

Waste piles: Noncontainerized accumulations of insoluble solid, nonflowing hazardous waste. Some waste piles are used for final disposal; many serve as temporary storage pending transfer of the waste to a final disposal site.

Land treatment: A disposal process in which solid waste, such as sludge from municipal sewage treatment plants, is applied onto

Table 6.4 Sources and estimated quantities of regulated medical wastes

Waste generator	Number of generators	Quantity produced (tons per year)
Hospitals	7,100	359,000
Long-term health-care facilities	12,700	29,600
Physicians' offices	180,000	26,400
Clinics	15,500	16,700
Laboratories	4,300	15,400
Dentists' offices	98,400	7,600
Veterinarians	38,000	4,600
Funeral homes	20,400	3,900
Freestanding blood banks	900	2,400
Total	377,300	465,600

Table 6.5 Types, regulation, and characteristics of commercially generated waste

Type of waste	Regulating body	Typical content	Approximate annual volume (1984)
Nonhazardous	State and local governments	Refuse, garbage, sludge, municipal trash	400 billion ft^3
Hazardous	EPA or authorized states	Solvents, acids, heavy metals, pesticide residues, chemical sludges, incinerator ash, plating solutions	4 billion ft^3 (1% of total)
Mixed	EPA and NRC or states	Radioactive organic liquids, radioactive heavy metals	60,000 ft^3 (0.00002% of total)
Radioactive	NRC or agreement states	High- and low-level radioactive waste, naturally occurring and accelerator-produced materials	3 million ft^3 (0.0007% of total)[a]

a. Commercial low-level radioactive waste only.

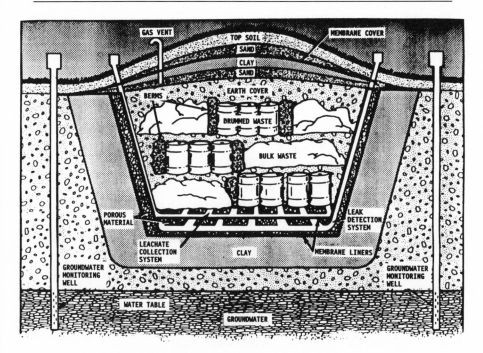

Figure 6.3   Land burial facility for hazardous waste

or incorporated in the soil surface. Microbes occurring naturally in the soil break down or immobilize the hazardous constituents. Land treatment facilities are also called land application or land farming facilities.

All approaches to disposing of hazardous wastes have potential impacts on public health and the environment. Improper discharge or burial on land has led to contamination of many supplies of groundwater, which serve as a source of drinking water. Such contamination can also subsequently move into streams, rivers, lakes, and other surface waters, killing aquatic life and destroying wildlife and vegetation. Incineration can produce airborne releases, and leachable heavy metal residues make disposal of the accompanying ash a problem. Nor are the harmful effects confined to inhalation or ingestion. Plastic fishing gear, six-pack-can beverage yokes, sandwich bags, and styrofoam cups thrown into the ocean entrap and kill more than 1 million seabirds and 100,000 marine mammals every year. In fact plastics may be as great a source of mortality to marine mammals as oil spills, heavy metals, or other toxic materials (Shea, 1988).

According to the EPA, the management of hazardous waste is probably our most serious environmental problem. The EPA strongly encourages producers to reduce the volume of hazardous waste by eliminating or minimizing their production, treating them onsite to render them nontoxic, or both (EPA, 1986b). Methods for minimizing the production of hazardous waste include:

Separating or segregating waste at its source to prevent hazardous materials from contaminating nonhazardous waste and thereby making the entire mixture hazardous

Recycling (recovery and reuse) through removal of hazardous materials from waste streams, reuse within the process (for example, recycling lead storage batteries), or transfer to another industry that can use the waste as input to its production process

Eliminating or substituting a raw material that generates little or no hazardous waste for one that generates a large amount (for example, the use of non-lead-based paints)

Changing manufacturing processes to eliminate steps that generate hazardous waste or altering processes so that the waste is no longer produced (for example, using more effective and efficient methods for applying paints)

Table 6.6 summarizes a range of techniques that can be used to reduce the volume of hazardous waste.

Several methods are available for treating hazardous waste before disposal. Such treatment usually takes place in tanks, surface impoundments, incinerators, and on land treatment facilities, but it can also be accomplished through processes such as distillation, centrifugation, reverse osmosis, ion exchange, and filtration. Because many of the treatment processes are waste-specific, the EPA has not attempted to develop detailed regulations for any particular type of process or equipment. Instead, it has established general requirements to assure safe containment. These requirements pertain primarily to avoiding equipment or process failure that could pose a hazard; for example, reagents that could cause equipment or a process to fail must not be used in treatment. In addition, safety systems to shut down inflow in case of a malfunction must be installed in continuous-flow operations (EPA, 1986a).

Table 6.6   Techniques for minimizing production of hazardous wastes

Inventory management and improved operations
Inventory and trace all raw materials
Emphasize use of nontoxic production materials
Provide waste minimization or reduction training for employees
Improve materials receiving, storage, and handling practices

Modification of equipment
Install equipment that produces minimal or no waste
Modify equipment to enhance recovery or recycling options
Redesign equipment or production lines to produce less waste
Improve operating efficiency of equipment
Maintain strict preventive maintenance program

Production process changes
Substitute nonhazardous for hazardous raw materials
Segregate wastes by type for recovery
Eliminate sources of leaks or spills
Separate hazardous from nonhazardous and radioactive from nonradioactive
    wastes
Redesign or reformulate end products to be less hazardous
Optimize reactions and raw material use

Recycling and reuse
Install closed-loop systems
Recycle onsite for reuse
Recycle offsite for reuse
Exchange wastes

Treatment to reduce toxicity and volume
Evaporation
Incineration
Compaction
Chemical conversion

Technologies that can be applied for the treatment of hazardous waste before disposal include (EPA, 1986a, 1986b):

Biological treatment using microorganisms to degrade organic compounds. Anaerobic bacteria capable of degrading and detoxifying polychlorinated biphenyls exist in nature; unfortunately, most waste disposal facilities are not designed to promote conditions that will favor the growth of microbes (Finstein, 1989).

Application of activated carbon to adsorb organic compounds from liquid waste. The problem of disposing of the contaminated carbon can be avoided if the adsorbed compounds are removed and recovered and the carbon reused.

Chemical treatment to neutralize acid or alkaline waste, to detoxify chlorinated substances, to oxidize and detoxify waste such as cyanides, phenols, and organic sulfur compounds, or to coagulate, precipitate, and concentrate suspended solids.

Solidification and stabilization of waste to make it less permeable and soluble and less susceptible to transport by water.

Incineration to destroy certain toxic chemicals or to make waste, particularly that containing organic compounds, less hazardous.

Cleanup of Existing Hazardous Waste Sites

There are thousands of hazardous waste disposal sites in the United States that were improperly designed or operated and have leaked, or have the potential to leak, hazardous waste into the environment. Recognizing the severity of the problem and the urgent need for cleanup of these sites, Congress passed the Superfund Act in 1980. Under its terms, the EPA designates sites for cleanup by including them in the National Priorities List. After a site has been listed, EPA identifies the potentially responsible parties and gives them an opportunity to implement cleanup. If they fail to do so, EPA arranges for the cleanup, using Superfund money, and then seeks to recover the costs from the responsible parties. Any owner, operator, transporter, or generator of hazardous waste can be held liable for the total costs for the cleanup of an existing site, regardless of the amount of waste the party deposited in it. The law imposes retroactive liability without time limitations. To obtain better information on industries that are using toxic chemicals and are therefore potential producers of hazardous waste, Title III of the Superfund Amendments and Reauthorization Act of 1986 requires industries to make public the chemicals and chemical hazards associated with their operations.

In addition to the sites contaminated by industrial waste, there is a host of sites contaminated by operations at various establishments of the U.S. Department of Defense (DOD) and Department of Energy (DOE). Many of the disposal sites created by DOE contain radioactive waste.

One approach used for the cleanup of hazardous waste sites is to dig up the contaminated material and transport it to a new burial site. Because in many cases the quantities of material are enormous, various methods for on-site treatment are being developed. Some of these involve mobile units that use biological, physical, chemical, and thermal technologies. Specific approaches include vapor extraction, solidification, soil flushing, vitrification, radio-frequency and direct-current heating, electrokinetics, and microbial degradation (Sims, 1990).

Benzene, toluene, xylenes, and other hazardous aromatic chemicals have been disposed in many land burial sites. These chemicals are also present in leakage from underground gasoline tanks. Field experience and research indicate that stabilization by biological organisms could play an important role in treating such wastes. This technique could be used on-site to oxidize these chemicals and many other hydrocarbons to nontoxic carbon dioxide and water, if the microorganisms are provided with necessary inorganic nutrients such as phosphate and ammonium nitrogen, plus oxygen (Abelson, 1986). However, any on-site treatment technique requires prior clearance from the EPA based on a detailed characterization of the site, including information on groundwater flow, the nature and distribution of the waste chemicals, their rate of movement in the site, and their potential for migration off the site.

Even though an array of processes has been proposed for the cleanup of hazardous waste sites, progress has been slow. Obstacles include the unproved nature of many of the proposed processes, the diversity of expertise required, the high costs, and the fact that no two sites are identical. Even within a single site, conditions may vary. Costs of cleanup range up to $1 million per acre, and some sites cover more than 100 acres. Where the groundwater has been contaminated, cleanup may take 20–40 years or even longer (Abelson, 1989).

Management and Disposal of Radioactive Waste

As is the case with hazardous chemical waste, the management and disposal of radioactive waste is receiving attention at all levels of government. The groups involved include Congress, the EPA, the U.S. Nuclear Regulatory Commission (NRC), DOE, and comparable agencies in many states, acting either alone or in regional compacts.

Table 6.7   Principal federal laws related to management and disposal
of radioactive waste

Year	Law	Public Law number
1954	Atomic Energy Act	85-703
1978	Uranium Mill Tailings Radiation Control Act	95-604
1980	Low-Level Radioactive Waste Policy Act	96-573
1983	Nuclear Waste Policy Act of 1982	97-425
1986	Low-Level Radioactive Waste Policy Amendments Act of 1985	99-240
1987	Nuclear Waste Policy Amendments Act	100-203

In general, Congress passes relevant legislation (Table 6.7), the EPA sets applicable environmental standards, and the NRC develops regulations to implement the standards. In the case of low-level radioactive waste, the states then arrange to have the necessary disposal facilities designed, constructed, and operated. In the case of high-level waste, Congress has made DOE responsible for the design, construction, and operation of suitable disposal facilities.

Table 6.8 summarizes the amounts and types of radioactive waste in temporary storage at various sites in the United States. These data represent the full range of waste, including uranium mill tailings, transuranic (chemical elements heavier than uranium) waste, waste

Table 6.8   Radioactive waste accumulated in the United States through 1988

Type of waste	Volume (m^3)	% of total	Activity (Curies)	% of total
Spent fuel	8.0×10^3	0.2	1.9×10^{10}	93.8
High-level	3.8×10^5	8.6	1.2×10^9	6.1
Low-level	3.8×10^6	84.9	1.8×10^7	0.1
Mill tailings	1.2×10^8	—	5.5×10^5	—
Transuranics	2.9×10^5	6.4	3.9×10^6	0.02

produced as a result of the decommissioning of nuclear power plants and related nuclear facilities, and waste from various remedial actions (cleanup of contaminated disposal facilities) and military activities. Figures from the National Research Council's Board on Radioactive Waste Management (BRWM) provide some perspective. Each 1,000-megawatt nuclear power plant annually produces about 30 tons of spent fuel, which if reprocessed and vitrified could be reduced to 4–11 cubic meters of high-level waste. Each such plant also produces some 100–300 cubic meters of short-lived low-level radioactive waste each year. In addition, the mining of uranium to provide fuel for each plant produces about 86,000 tons of mill tailings annually (BRWM, 1990). Additional low-level waste is produced by the use of radioactive material in medicine, research, and industry.

Low-Level Waste

Over 80 percent of the total volume of radioactive waste generated in the United States is low-level. Although it contains much less than 1 percent of the total quantity of radionuclides being disposed of, its annual volume in 1990 was 1.5 million cubic feet. Commercial nuclear power plants account for more than half of this volume and for over 80 percent of the total activity in such waste (Figure 6.4).

In the past, the approach commonly used to dispose of low-level radioactive waste was shallow land burial. Although this is similar to the approach used for hazardous (nonradioactive) chemical waste, there are basic differences. Whereas the EPA regulations for hazardous waste require a double liner and leachate monitoring system, the NRC regulations for low-level radioactive waste focus more on the waste form and packaging and specify a disposal facility design that minimizes the need for active maintenance (NRC, 1982). Consequently, generators of mixed waste (containing both radioactive material and hazardous chemicals) face the dilemma of complying with contradictory EPA and NRC regulations. Compounding this dilemma, EPA regulations forbid interim storage of mixed waste and are somewhat vague about the quantity of toxic chemicals that must be present in low-level radioactive waste to make it "hazardous." Efforts are being made to resolve the differences in the regulations of the two agencies.

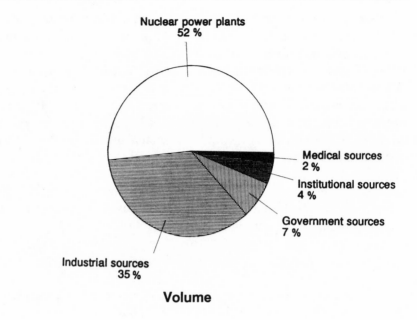

Volume

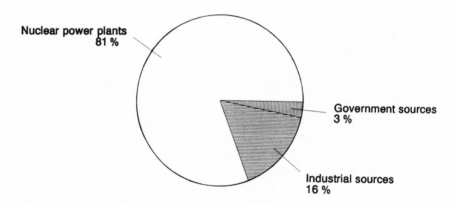

Activity

Figure 6.4   Relative volume and radionuclide content (activity) in low-level radioactive wastes from various sources

With the formation of state compacts to develop low-level radioactive waste disposal sites, there has been a shift away from shallow land burial as the primary method of disposal. A major impetus for this change has been public demand for disposal methods that provide greater safety and security. As a result, a variety of alternatives, each judged to be superior, is being proposed. These range from above- and below-ground vaults to earth-mounded concrete bunkers (Figure 6.5). Undoubtedly still more disposal options and modifications will be developed.

High-Level Waste

The principal sources of high-level radioactive waste are the operation of nuclear power plants and programs of DOD and DOE. Such waste includes spent (used) fuel removed from nuclear plants, and fission products separated from military fuel that has been chemically processed. In the latter case the unused uranium remaining in the fuel and the newly formed plutonium are reclaimed for reuse. In the United States, where commercial nuclear power plant fuel is no longer chemically processed, the spent fuel removed from such facilities is being stored on-site until a geologic repository for its disposal can be completed. In countries such as France, Germany, Japan, and the

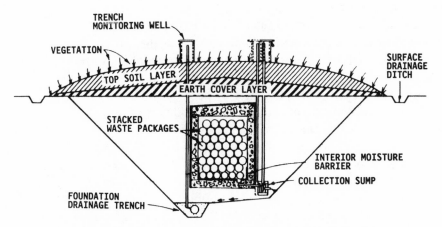

Figure 6.5   Earth-mounded concrete bunker for disposal of low-level radioactive wastes

United Kingdom, where spent fuel from commercial nuclear plants is being chemically processed, the fission products, initially separated out as liquid waste, are subsequently solidified and held for ultimate disposal in a geologic repository.

Through the Nuclear Waste Policy Act of 1982 and the Nuclear Waste Policy Amendments Act of 1987, Congress took what it considered to be positive steps to solve the high-level radioactive waste disposal problem. The program initiated by these laws has three essential components: (1) design and construction of a geologic repository for permanent disposal of spent fuel and other high-level waste, (2) establishment of a "monitored retrievable storage" (MRS) facility for temporary storage and packaging of spent fuel prior to placement in a repository, and (3) development of a transportation system for moving the waste from its source to the MRS facility and ultimately to the repository. Congress also specified that initial studies for a high-level waste repository be limited to the Yucca Mountain site in Nevada.

The standards developed by the EPA for the high-level waste repository are probabilistic in nature and include the following key stipulations (EPA, 1991):

For the first 10,000 years after disposal, projected releases of radioactive material to the environment from the repository will cause no more than 1,000 premature cancer deaths per 100,000 metric tons of heavy-metal waste. This amount of waste is comparable to what will be produced by the existing nuclear power plants in the United States over their projected operating lifetime. Compliance with this objective will assure that the public health risk from the waste placed in the repository will be no greater than that which would have been present if the uranium ore giving rise to the waste had not been mined.

For the first 10,000 years after disposal, cumulative releases to the accessible environment shall have a likelihood of less than 1 chance in 10 of exceeding the quantities for certain radionuclides specified in the standards, and less than 1 chance in 1,000 of exceeding 10 times the specified quantities. Compliance with these objectives will assure that the limit on premature cancer deaths is not exceeded.

Annual doses to members of the public shall not exceed 0.25 millisievert (25 millirem) to the whole body (see Chapter 9). These requirements apply to the *undisturbed* performance of the repository for 1,000 years after disposal of the waste.

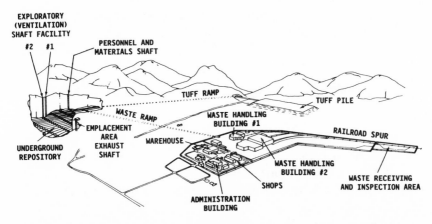

EXPLORATORY
(VENTILATION)
SHAFT FACILITY

#2   #1

PERSONNEL AND
MATERIALS SHAFT

TUFF RAMP

TUFF PILE

WASTE RAMP

WASTE HANDLING
BUILDING #1

EMPLACEMENT
AREA

RAILROAD SPUR

WAREHOUSE

UNDERGROUND
REPOSITORY

EXHAUST
SHAFT

WASTE HANDLING
BUILDING #2

WASTE RECEIVING
AND INSPECTION AREA

SHOPS

ADMINISTRATION
BUILDING

Figure 6.6   Proposed geologic repository in Yucca Mountain, Nevada, for
disposal of high-level radioactive wastes

In developing regulations for assuring compliance with the EPA
standards, the NRC imposed the following requirements on DOE:
the repository must be designed so that the waste can be retrieved;
containment of the waste must be "substantially complete" for
300–1,000 years or more after repository closure; subsequent release
rates from the waste must not exceed certain limits; the groundwater
travel time from the repository to the accessible environment must be
at least 1,000 years; and both the geologic repository operations area
and the controlled area must be located on lands under the jurisdiction
and control of the federal government (NRC, 1981). Figure 6.6 is a
schematic diagram of the repository being proposed for the Yucca
Mountain site.

On the basis of these requirements, DOE is conducting studies to
determine whether the proposed Yucca Mountain site meets the basic
technical and legal requirements. The key questions being evaluated
are:

What can happen? A range of scenarios is being developed for
various possible events in the repository under both normal and
accident conditions.

How likely is it? The probabilities of occurrence are estimated for
each postulated event.

What are the consequences? Models are being developed for estimating the radionuclide releases that might occur, the pathways by which they might cause exposure of the public, and the associated risks.

Are the postulated events and consequences acceptable? The estimated risks for the repository are compared with NRC regulations and EPA standards.

If the data indicate that the Yucca Mountain site can safely isolate high-level wastes, the Nuclear Waste Policy Act requires that DOE, with presidential approval, apply to the NRC for a license to construct a repository. The NRC will then determine whether the proposed site meets federal regulations; if it does, construction can begin. Although there have been many delays in developing plans for the repository, the target date for initial emplacement of high-level waste is 2010.

Incineration of Radioactive and Hazardous Waste

Incineration is one of several technologies available both for reducing the volume of solid and hazardous waste and for destroying certain toxic chemicals in it. With the increased use of plastics in packaging, however, there has been a corresponding increase in the amount of polyvinyl chloride in solid waste. When burned, such plastics produce hydrochloric acid. This extremely corrosive compound can destroy incinerator components, such as metal heat exchangers and flue-gas scrubbers, and can threaten human health if released into the atmosphere. Hydrochloric acid can also be produced in incinerators by the combustion of foods and other waste containing chloride salts.

Compounding these problems, incomplete combustion of some organic materials in the presence of chlorides can produce dioxins, a toxic group of compounds. Dioxins may be present in the airborne emissions from the incinerator as well as in the solid residues. However, if the operating temperature of the incinerator is sufficiently high, and if there are adequate distribution and mixing of the combustion air, production of these compounds can be avoided or reduced to very low levels. In fact EPA studies of airborne dioxin emissions from five municipal waste incinerators showed that the amounts released did not constitute a health hazard to people living in the immediate vicinity. Other studies, however, have failed to support these findings. As a result, more research is needed (Engdahl, Barrett, and Trayser, 1986).

Key factors in avoiding unwanted products are the incinerator's operating temperature and the retention time for the waste at maximum temperature. Because many solid wastes yield little heat during combustion, achieving the desired temperature may be difficult without the use of supplementary fuels. New approaches, however, are being developed to overcome these problems. One possibility is to locate incinerators on oceangoing vessels to burn the waste offshore at some distance from population groups.

These potential threats to human health have led to stringent regulations limiting emissions from incinerator facilities. Although modern technology will provide almost any degree of cleanup required, the economic costs can be high. One response has been to construct and operate centrally located incinerators to serve a group of waste producers. In many communities that, for environmental, political, economic, and other reasons, have a limited capacity for the direct disposal of solid wastes in landfills, incineration has become the principal method of intermediate treatment. A wide range of incinerators can be used for this purpose. Figure 6.7 shows the most common type.

Although the technology is available to control their airborne emissions, use of incinerators has lagged because of public opposition and misunderstanding. In the case of low-level radioactive waste, this delay is especially unfortunate because incinerators appear to be one of the best available pretreatment technologies. In 1990 there were fully licensed and operational incinerators at four nuclear power plant sites that had either never been operated or had undergone only limited testing and then been shut down (Long, 1990). Another factor contributing to the delay is the relatively low cost of disposing of untreated (compacted or noncompacted) low-level radioactive waste in land-burial facilities. This situation, however, appears to be changing rapidly.

Although finding a place to dispose of ash from the incineration of hazardous or low-level radioactive waste might be difficult, the ash represents a much better form for burial than the original waste: it is biologically and structurally more stable, and many of the compounds it contains are insoluble (Long, 1990). Incineration would also produce a waste that minimizes long-term ground subsidence and leaching by rain and groundwater.

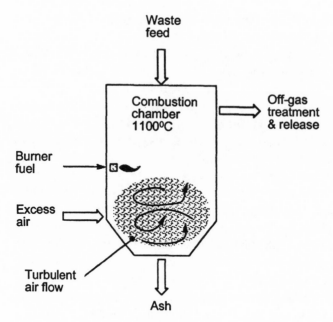

Figure 6.7   Excess-air incinerator with vertical furnace (single-stage cyclone)

Addressing Public Concerns

Though still maturing, incineration is an effective and advanced technology with tremendous potential for intermediate treatment (volume
reduction) of solid, hazardous, and low-level radioactive wastes. Nev-
ertheless, public concern persists about possible environmental damage from the release of toxic materials in the ash and the off-gases.
Another concern often voiced is that an incineration or land burial
facility will add truck traffic and reduce property values in the surrounding community. For these reasons, sites for such facilities
should be located away from residential and highly populated areas.

This "not-in-my-backyard" syndrome extends to the siting of pris-
ons, airports, mental health centers, and power plants. Unfortunately,
the talented people responsible for the design, construction, and operation of such facilities rarely know how to deal with such concerns.
According to one group of experts, workable, legitimate sitings of
waste treatment and disposal facilities will require: (1) a comprehensive, integrated management strategy giving primary emphasis to

waste reduction, detoxification, and recycling; (2) extensive interactive participation by citizens, regulators, and waste managers during planning, siting, and operations; and (3) new institutional arrangements and guarantees that instill public confidence in the need for and safety of proposed facilities. Those attempting to develop such a program should understand the serious concerns of people who oppose waste disposal facilities: regulatory officials' apparent lack of enforcement, public health agencies' refusals to negotiate or to take local concerns seriously, government's failure to clean up known toxic waste sites that remain hazardous, state organizations' and industry's "closed" information policies, continual underestimations of the public's ability to comprehend issues, and a lack of good-faith efforts to involve citizens in the process (Peelle and Ellis, 1987).

A variety of principles, observations, and tactics can be used to minimize or overcome these perceptions (Connor, 1988). One is to realize that the main sources of public concern are perceived risks and inequities, threats to community integrity, and improper or arbitrary decision making. Information and consultation must begin early in the project and continue through the environmental assessment process. Perceptions of inequity often arise when the benefits of a facility will be highly diffused but the drawbacks will be concentrated; in some cases, some form of compensation for the affected groups may be appropriate. If the proposed facility threatens major changes in the local landscape or an influx of outsiders, involving local residents in the initial development of the project offers a constructive outlet for expressing and responding to their concerns. Perceptions of improper or arbitrary decision making arise primarily when engineers make decisions on issues which they believe to be purely technical and professional, but which the people affected view as issues of political power. When possible, residents should be given a voice, particularly in the development of criteria for site selection.

It is also important to realize that the "public" is not one homogeneous group. It includes not only local residents but also suppliers, unions, and regulators. It is vital to identify these groups at the outset, to ascertain what they know and believe about the project, and to ensure that they receive the information they need. It it also important that project developers and regulators have adequate information about local channels of communication, views on growth, knowledge of and attitudes toward the industry involved, the developer of the

Table 6.9   Relation of public participation to success in establishment of waste disposal facilities

Public participation	Project outcomes	
	Successful	Unsuccessful
Agency "sells" premade decision		●
Agency redefines public demand or concern		●
No prior public education efforts		●
Public hearings		●
Agency seeks public-attitude data	●	
Agency seeks public-needs data	●	
Workshops or small group meetings	●	
Prior public education efforts	●	
Agency exchanges written information with public groups	●	

project, and the project itself. How these issues are addressed will play a key role in the establishment of any type of waste management and disposal facility. Close, frequent, and proper interaction with local groups can lead to a successful project; improper interactions will almost assuredly lead to failure (Table 6.9).

In the final analysis, the important fact to know is whether improper disposal of hazardous waste is harming people. A survey of sites on the EPA National Priorities List has furnished some interesting data on this subject (U.S. Department of Health and Human Services, 1990). More than 4 million people lived within one mile of the 725 sites for which data were available. Young children, women of childbearing age, and elderly persons accounted for almost 50 percent of this total. A review of 951 sites showed documented evidence of migration of metals at 34 percent, and of volatile organic chemicals at 28 percent. In approximately three-quarters of these sites, the groundwater had been contaminated. Although methods for determining health effects on the potentially affected populations are limited and more research is needed, consultations identified eye irritation, dermatologic effects, respiratory problems, and a variety of neurological complaints as the most commonly reported adverse effects. Conditions and exposure potentials at 109 of the 951 sites were considered to constitute ongoing or probable public health concerns; conditions and exposure potentials at 803 sites were considered to represent possible public health concerns.

The General Outlook

Most current procedures for disposing of hazardous and radioactive waste involve land burial, ranging from near the surface for hazardous and low-level radioactive waste to deep underground for high-level radioactive waste. Given that much chemical waste will remain toxic for hundreds of thousands of years, and that certain high-level radioactive waste will require thousands of years to decay, it is a matter of urgent necessity to develop methods for reducing or eliminating generation of this waste or for converting it into less hazardous material. Chemical reprocessing of spent fuel from nuclear power plants, currently practiced in other industrial nations but not in the United States, would represent an advance in dealing with high-level radioactive waste. Recycling the separated plutonium and reclaimed uranium as fuel in other nuclear power plants would convert the long-lived and hazardous plutonium to less hazardous and shorter-lived fission products.

As in the case of air, water, and food contamination, a systems approach is essential in the evaluation and analysis of this environmental problem. For example, one approach being used to reduce airborne emissions from major coal-burning plants is to install scrubbers. However, not only do scrubbers reduce electrical output, but the sulfur dioxide removal process produces large volumes of solid waste. An alternative is to push forward with the development of new clean coal-burning technologies, such as the integrated gasification combined-cycle technology, that promise to eliminate many of these problems (Abelson, 1990). The gas produced by this process can be used to make liquid fuel or can be burned directly to generate electricity. The residue from the coal takes the form of a glassy impervious frit that should be readily amenable to disposal; for example, it can be used as a substitute for crushed stone or aggregate.

Although industrial operations are a major source of solid waste in the United States, consumer activities also make a sizable contribution, in the form of discarded clothing, yard debris, plastic packaging, and an estimated 16 billion disposable diapers, 1.6 billion pens, and 2 billion razors each year (Langone, 1989). Our favorite consumer products, automobiles, account for more than 200 million worn-out tires per year, as well as tons of waste metal (which fortunately can be recycled), lead batteries, brake linings that may be toxic, and air-conditioning refrigerant (whose release to the atmosphere may lead to destruction of the ozone layer) (Herman, Siamak, and Ausubel, 1989).

The declining number of municipal landfills highlights the importance of reducing the volume of all types of solid waste. To reduce the volume of domestic waste, the EPA is considering establishing an immediate goal of recycling 45–50 percent of the wastes produced by American householders (Donahue, 1988). A $400 million plant is being constructed to recycle up to 45 percent of the newsprint in New York City. And there is a ready market for recycled materials such as aluminum and glass. Major problems have developed, however, with respect to the recycling of plastics. Some 46 different resins, often in combination, are in common use in the manufacture of plastics. Few recycling processes can handle more than one type. Most current recycling activity is centered on polyethylene teraphthalate (PET), the material found in soft-drink bottles, and high-density polyethylene (HDPE), found in milk and motor-oil bottles (Fine, 1989; Shea, 1988).

Using biodegradable plastics may help, but for the long term other approaches are needed. These include changing our industrial processes to eliminate such materials, developing more methods for recycling, and discovering ways to use waste material beneficially instead of burying it. An excellent example of this last approach is the current use of discarded plastics as substitutes for other materials, such as wood, metal, or glass. For example, processes have been developed for converting plastics into synthetic wood that is resistant to water, corrosion, chemicals, bacteria, and insects (Brown, 1989). In the final analysis, there is only so much land where such materials can be buried, and groundwater sources, once contaminated, may be lost for thousands of years. The disposal of solid wastes is a problem of enormous magnitude. Solving it will require changes both in our technology and in our lifestyles.

REFERENCES

Abelson, Philip H. 1986. "Treatment of Hazardous Wastes." Editorial. *Science* 233, no. 4763 (1 August), 509.
—— 1989. "Cleaning Hazardous Waste Sites." Editorial. *Science* 246, no. 4934 (1 December), 1097.
—— 1990. "New Technology for Cleaner Air." Editorial. *Science* 248, no. 4957 (18 May), 793.
Brown, Sandford. 1989. "A Big Pickup in Plastics." *The Lamp* 71, no. 4 (Winter), 24–29.
BRWM. 1990. *Rethinking High-Level Radioactive Waste Disposal.* Washington, D.C.: National Academy Press.
Connor, D. M. 1988. "Breaking Through the 'NIMBY' Syndrome." *Civil Engineering* 58, no. 12 (December), 69–72.
Council for Solid Waste Solutions. 1989. "The Urgent Need to Recycle." Special advertising section, *Time,* 17 July.
Donahue, Christine. 1988. "Waking Up to the Hot Issue of the 1990s: Garbage." *Adweek's Marketing Week,* 28 November, pp. 57–59.
Engdahl, R. B., R. E. Barrett, and D. A. Trayser. 1986. "Process Emissions and Their Control: Part I." In *Air Pollution, Supplement to Measurements, Monitoring, Surveillance, and Engineering Control,* ed. A. C. Stern. 3d ed. New York: Academic Press.
EPA. 1982. "Environmental Radiation Protection Standards for the Management and Disposal of Spent Nuclear Fuel, High-Level and Transuranic Radioactive Waste." Title 40, Part 191, Code of Federal Regulations.
—— 1986a. *RCRA Orientation Manual.* Report EPA/530-SW-86-001. Washington, D.C.
—— 1986b. *Solving the Hazardous Waste Problem: EPA's RCRA Program.* Report EPA/530-SW-86-037. Washington, D.C.
—— 1989. *The Toxics-Release Inventory: A National Perspective.* Report EPA 560/4-89-005. Washington, D.C.
—— 1990. *Medical Waste Management in the United States.* First Interim Report to Congress. Washington, D.C.
—— 1991. "Environmental Radiation Protection Standards for the Management and Disposal of Spent Nuclear Fuel, High-Level and Transuranic Radioactive Waste." Title 40, Part 191, Code of Federal Regulations (Draft Revised Standards).
Fine, Susan. 1989. "The Nine Lives of Plastic." *World-Watch* 2, no. 3 (May–June), 43–44.
Finstein, M. S. 1989. "Composting Solid Waste: Costly Mismanagement of a Microbial Ecosystem." *American Society for Microbiology News* 55, no. 11 (November), 599–602.

Herman, Robert, Siamak A. Ardekani, and Jessie H. Ausubel. 1989. "Dematerialization." In *Technology and Environment,* ed. Jesse H. Ausubel and Hedy E. Sladovich. Washington, D.C.: National Academy Press.

Langone, John. 1989. "Waste: A Stinking Mess." *Time,* 2 January, pp. 44, 45, and 47.

Linnerooth, Joanne, and Allen V. Kneese. 1989. "Hazardous Waste Management: A West German Approach." *Resources,* no. 96 (Summer), 7–10.

Long, S. W. 1990. *The Incineration of Low-Level Radioactive Waste.* Report NUREG-1393. Washington, D.C.: U.S. Nuclear Regulatory Commission.

NRC. 1981. "Disposal of High-Level Radioactive Wastes in Geologic Repositories." Title 10, Part 60, Code of Federal Regulations.

——— 1982. "Licensing Requirements for Land Disposal of Radioactive Waste." Title 10, Part 61, Code of Federal Regulations.

——— 1990. *Information Digest, 1990 Edition.* Vol. 2. Report NUREG-1350. Washington, D.C.

Peelle, E., and R. Ellis. 1987. "Beyond the 'Not-in-My-Backyard' Impasse." *Forum for Applied Research and Public Policy* 2, no. 3, pp. 68–77.

Shea, Cynthia. 1988. "Plastic Waste Proliferates." *World-Watch* 1, no. 2 (March–April), 7–8.

Sims, Ronald C. 1990. "Soil Remediation Techniques at Uncontrolled Hazardous Waste Sites: A Critical Review." *Journal of the Air & Waste Management Association* 40, no. 5 (May), 704–732.

U.S. Department of Health and Human Services. 1990. *ATSDR Biennial Report to Congress.* Vol. 7. Atlanta: Agency for Toxic Substances and Disease Registry.

7

Rodents and Insects

Scientists estimate that there are 10 million insect species in the world (Holden, 1989). Some of these, such as the honeybee and silkworm, bring financial benefits; others, such as the butterfly and lightning bug, are aesthetically pleasing. Still others, however, such as flies, mosquitoes, boll weevils, corn borers, termites, and locusts, are destructive and even dangerous to humans. The mosquito, in particular, is the vector (transmitter) for a wide range of disease agents. The common housefly is also thought to be implicated in a number of human diseases.

Rodents are also known to be transmitters of disease agents and represent a major challenge to environmental health. It is estimated that in the United States there are 125 million rats, or 1 for every 2 people. Table 7.1 lists the diseases that can be transmitted by rodents and various insects. These diseases continue to have major public health, social, and economic impacts throughout the world.

Rodents

Rodents have been a public health problem for centuries. Most famous is the role of rats in the successive epidemics of bubonic plague, called collectively the Black Death, that swept Europe in the fourteenth century. One of the earliest recorded epidemics was launched in 1347 in Genoa, when ships arriving from Black Sea ports brought rats carrying infected fleas (Duplaix, 1988). The subsequent spread of bubonic plague depopulated some 200,000 towns and in three years killed some 25 million people, or a quarter of the population in Europe. The Black Death remains the greatest calamity in human history. In 1665 another epidemic of plague killed 100,000 people in London; in

Table 7.1 Public health impact of various insects and rodents

Vector	Impact
Flies	Diarrhea, dysentery, conjunctivitis, typhoid, cholera, fly larvae infestations, annoyances
Mosquitoes	Encephalitis, malaria, yellow fever (urban), dengue, filariasis, annoyances, bites
Lice	Epidemic typhus, louse-borne relapsing fever, trench fever, bites, annoyances
Fleas	Plague, endemic typhus, bites, annoyances
Mites	Scabies, rickettsial pox, scrub typhus, bites, annoyances
Ticks	Lyme disease, tick paralysis, tick-borne relapsing fever, Rocky Mountain spotted fever, tularemia, bites, annoyances
Bedbugs, kissing bugs	Bites, annoyances, Chagas' disease
Ants	Bites, annoyances
Rodents	Rat-bite fever, leptospirosis, salmonellosis, rat bites

the 1890s it struck in San Francisco; and today it continues to exist in Africa, Asia, and both North and South America.

Characteristics

Rodents are believed to be the fastest-reproducing mammals. Their gestation period is 21–25 days, and they can reproduce every 60–90 days. A typical litter size ranges from five to nine. Their life span is 9–12 months.

Rats are very intelligent and survive in a hostile human environment by means of complex social mechanisms. They have a keen sense of smell, like the same food as people, and prefer it fresh. Rats have a well-developed sense of touch through the nose, whiskers, and hair. They also have an excellent sense of balance and can fall three stories without injury. All rats are accomplished swimmers. Rats can also eat decayed food and consume contaminated water with no apparent ill effects.

Rats are seldom seen in the daytime. They are cowardly and will seldom pick a fight. They follow established paths, which are readily identified by the presence of droppings (feces), urine stains (located by using ultraviolet light), and their characteristic odor (Fischer, 1969).

Rats are extremely adaptable and can survive under very adverse conditions (Canby, 1977; Lore and Flannelly, 1977). Scientists returning to Pacific islands that were virtually destroyed in nuclear weapons tests in the early 1950s found flourishing colonies of rats. The same species that lives in burrows in the United States and in attics in Europe can live in palm trees in the South Pacific. Other species, finding shortages of food on land, have learned to dive into lakes and ponds to catch fish.

Three species of rodents cause major environmental concern in the United States today: the Norway rat, the roof rat, and the house mouse. Species of importance in other parts of the world include the Polynesian rat (*Rattus exulans*), which has spread from its native Southeast Asia to New Zealand and Hawaii; and the lesser bandicoot (*Bandicota bengalensis*), which is predominant in southern Asia, especially India. The main impact of these rodents is their widespread destruction of food, particularly grains (Canby, 1977).

Knowing the characteristics of the rodents that pose an environmental problem is essential to their control. Figure 7.1 highlights the anatomic differences of the most common rodents in the United States.

The Norway rat (*Rattus norvegicus*): characterized by its relatively large size and shorter tail. Norway rats frequent the lower parts of buildings and occupy harborages in woodpiles, rubbish, and debris. They also burrow under floors, concrete slabs, and footings and live around residences, warehouses, chicken yards, and in sewers. They nest in the ground and have a range of 100–150 feet.

The roof rat (*Rattus rattus*): characterized by its smaller size and longer tail. Roof rats live in grain mills, dense growth in willows, and old residential neighborhoods. They are excellent climbers, frequently occupying shrubbery, trees, and the upper parts of buildings. They usually nest in buildings and have a range similar to that of the Norway rat.

The house mouse (*Mus musculus*): characterized by its small size,

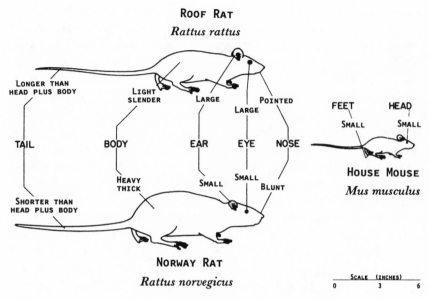

ROOF RAT

Rattus rattus

HOUSE MOUSE

Mus musculus

NORWAY RAT

Rattus norvegicus

SCALE (INCHES)

Figure 7.1   Anatomic characteristics of three species of rodents

including small feet and eyes, and long tail. Mice live in buildings and in fields. Their effects are primarily of a nuisance nature. Since their range is limited (10–30 feet), these effects are localized. They will not be discussed further.

Impacts

Rats affect the quality of life in many ways. Although their ability to transmit disease is important, they also have significant economic impacts and social implications.

Public Health Impacts

In addition to bubonic plague, rats can transmit typhus fever through infected fleas, salmonellosis through food contaminated by their urine, and rat-bite fever through a spirochete in their blood. In poor housing conditions, infants, paraplegics, and people under the influence of alcohol or drugs are especially vulnerable to rat bites. On babies, the targets for mutilation are often the nose, ears, lips, fingers, and toes.

Economic Impacts

One rat can eat 10 bushels of grain or 40 pounds of food per year. Rats are estimated to destroy 20 percent of the world's crops each year, including 48 million tons of growing rice and some 30–40 million tons of bread grains and rice in storage. In places like India, they represent serious competition to humans for food. In the United States rats are estimated to cause about $1 billion in losses per year. This figure includes fires caused by rodents chewing on electrical wiring. In fact 25 percent of fires in rural areas are estimated to be caused by rodents (Canby, 1977).

Social Implications

To many inner-city residents, the presence of rats is a vivid and gruesome symptom of community environmental degradation, a token of the larger pattern of social and economic breakdown and disorder in the real world of the urban poor. The appalling quality of life in such conditions often becomes clear to others only during projects for urban renewal, when rats from buildings that are being torn down or renovated stream into adjacent neighborhoods.

Control

One of the earliest accounts of attempts at rodent control dates to 1284, when the now-legendary Pied Piper of Hamelin played on his pipe and led all the rats in the town into the river Weser, where they drowned (Guest, 1984). Rodent control is complex because it is so closely tied to human behavior and to large-scale social and economic factors. Effective control programs, however, are possible; they consist of the following three basic elements.

Eliminating Food Sources

Rats cannot live and reproduce without food. Making food unavailable to them requires control of garbage and refuse, which in turn requires comprehensive public education. Garbage must be stored in metal cans with tight-fitting lids and should be collected twice a week; otherwise, storage containers will be filled, and residents will switch to plastic bags or cardboard boxes, which rats can easily tear open. Steps must also be taken to prevent accumulation of solid waste, which can provide harborage for rats, and to eliminate readily accessible sources of water such as dripping faucets.

Ratproofing

Ratproofing of buildings is an essential part of a long-range control program. Existing buildings should be modified so that rats cannot enter or leave, buildings that cannot be ratproofed should be demolished, and strict codes should be enacted to assure proper construction of new buildings.

Ratproofing existing buildings involves sealing all openings and installing a concrete floor or underground shields outside the building walls to prevent rats from burrowing underneath; a young rat can squeeze through a ½-inch opening, and a young mouse through a ¼-inch hole.

Traps, Fumigants, or Poisons

Once all buildings have been ratproofed and food has been made unavailable, the rat population can be reduced by trapping, fumigation, or poisoning programs inside buildings and areawide kills outdoors.

Traps avoid the use of poisons, but the rats that are caught must be collected and buried or incinerated. In the process, their fleas may be transferred to people.

Fumigants consist of gases, such as calcium cyanide and methyl bromide, that are released inside buildings. They provide a quick kill but require care to prevent dangerous exposures to people during use.

Poisons are generally placed in food (baits) for the rats. Examples include:

• Warfarin: a slow-acting anticoagulant rodenticide. Unfortunately, many rats have developed immunity to this chemical.

- Red squill: a bitter-tasting red powder that causes heart paralysis. It is effective only for the Norway rat.
- Zinc phosphide: a fast-acting black powder with a garlic odor that reacts with acid in the rat's stomach to produce phosphine gas. Most animals are repelled by it, but rats relish it.
- Norbormide: a fast-acting poison that causes shock impairment of blood circulation. It too is lethal only to Norway rats.

Effective use of rat poisons, however, is difficult. Rats have developed efficient feeding strategies that enable the members of a colony to avoid poisoned baits and to adjust to sudden changes in the food supply. Both laboratory and wild rats tend to avoid any contact with novel objects in their environment. Typically they avoid a new food for several days, and they may never sample it if the existing diet is nutritionally adequate. Eventually, small sublethal quantities of the new food may be ingested. If feeding animals become sick, the entire colony thereafter avoids the new food. This phenomenon, called conditioned food aversion, has forced psychologists to revise some basic principles of learning theory and has generated a lively interest in how animals acquire biologically meaningful information. It takes many trials to teach a hungry rat to press a bar for a food reward, and the rat never learns the trick unless the food is made available immediately after the bar is pressed. In contrast, a rat learns to avoid poisoned food in a single trial, even though it may not become sick until several hours after eating (Lore and Flannelly, 1977).

Other approaches being developed or considered for rat control include ultrasonic generators, single-dose chemosterilants that could sterilize both male and female rats, and new rodenticides that are rat-specific and thus not hazardous to nontarget animals.

Insects

As with rodents, the control of insects requires knowledge of their characteristics, including their life cycles and breeding habits, as well as their role in transmitting agents of disease.

Characteristics

Insects are highly specialized. Houseflies, for example, have hundreds of eyes mounted in such a way as to provide them with wide-range vision, coupled with unusual visual acuity. Some insects can detect sex attractants more than 15 miles away. An ant can lift 50 times its weight (Conniff, 1977).

The life cycles of the group of insects that includes mosquitoes and flies consist of four stages: egg, larva, pupa, and adult. Many insects lay hundreds or thousands of eggs, and some pass through their entire life cycle in a matter of days or weeks, producing numerous generations each season. A tiny fraction surviving the winter can quickly multiply to enormous numbers in the spring.

Some dark-colored insects survive cold weather by absorbing sunlight. Others absorb heat by basking on dark surfaces, or have heavy layers of hair or scales that retard heat loss. Some can beat their wings to keep warm while at rest. Still others survive subfreezing temperatures by lowering the freezing point of their body fluids, producing compounds that function similarly to the antifreeze used in automobile radiators. For example, in midwinter as much as 35 percent of the body weight of the eastern tent caterpillar may be glycerol; by spring, the glycerol has all but disappeared. Other insects protect themselves by purging their body fluids of nucleators, tiny specks of dust to which other molecules (such as ice) can attach, before hibernating for the winter (Conniff, 1977).

Impacts

Each year insects infect millions of people with diverse agents of disease (Table 7.2). Mosquitoes alone cause more than 250 million new cases of malaria worldwide (Hoffman et al., 1991). In Africa alone, this disease causes an estimated 1 to 2 million deaths (mostly of children) annually (Holden, 1989). An estimated 90 million people have lymphatic filariasis, an infection caused by a parasitic worm transmitted by mosquitoes. In fact filariasis is one of the most rapidly spreading diseases. Various kinds of flies can also be major transmitters of disease agents. For example, the World Health Organization estimates that there are 17 million cases of onchocerciasis, or river blindness, mostly in Africa. This disease is initiated by infective larvae passed through the bite of the black fly. As of 1990 at least 300,000 people had lost their vision as a result of onchocerciasis (American Public Health Association, 1990).

Although insect-related diseases are not as prevalent in the United

States as in most other countries, they represent an important public health problem. Each year several hundred people die from insect stings or from vectorborne diseases such as encephalitis or Rocky Mountain spotted fever; and tens of thousands suffer illness or injury from insect bites. Moreover, the situation is constantly changing; for example, Lyme disease has recently become a major concern in certain areas of the United States. On the east coast and in the northern great plains, this disease is spread by the bite of the *Ixodes dammini* tick; in the western states it is transmitted by the bite of the *Ixodes pacificus* tick. Both are common parasites of deer and mice. Because young stages of these ticks are only as large as a poppy seed, they often go undetected on humans. The first cluster of cases of Lyme disease was reported in Connecticut in 1975; it is now known to be present in over 40 states (Weinstein, 1990), and more than 8,000 new cases are reported each year (Spielman, 1991).

Insects have an enormous economic impact on agricultural production. They attack all stages of plant life, eating seeds, seedlings, roots, stems, leaves, flowers, and fruit; after the harvest, they eat the stored product. In the United States insects destroy an estimated 13 percent of agricultural crops (Holden, 1989); in Tanzania they destroy an estimated 25 percent; in Kenya, an estimated 75 percent. Insects also eat wooden buildings and woolen clothing. In many parts of the world, the persistent biting of mosquitoes, black flies, and other bloodsucking insects seriously impairs the productive capacity of workers, some-

Table 7.2   Global impacts of tropical disease infections

Disease	Insect vector	Number of countries affected	Number of people infected (millions)	Total population at risk (millions)
Malaria	Mosquitoes	103	270	2,100
Lymphatic filariasis	Mosquitoes	76	90	900
River blindness	Black flies	34	17	90
Chagas' disease	Triatomine (kissing bugs)	21	16–18	90
Leishmaniasis	Sandflies	80	12	350

times even bringing work to a standstill. Infestations of bedbugs, lice, and mites also cause persistent discomfort and disease.

Because of the widespread presence of mosquitoes and flies, this chapter focuses on problems associated with these two groups of insects.

Mosquitoes

Essentially every person in the world has heard the buzzing and suffered the bites of mosquitoes. Their characteristics, especially in their interactions with humans, may provide the key to their control.

Characteristics

Though seemingly frail, mosquitoes show remarkable abilities in flight: those that fly during the day navigate by polarized light from the sun; those that fly at night navigate by the stars. Their wings move even faster than a hummingbird's—an estimated 250–600 strokes per second (Conniff, 1977)—and produce the familiar whine that serves as their mating call. In general, however, mosquitoes do not fly when the temperature is below 57°F (14°C); they seldom fly at altitudes greater than several thousand feet; and their maximum flying speed is 7 miles per hour. As a result, they cannot maneuver if the wind is greater than 8 miles per hour. In fact winds disrupt the zigzag flight patterns that mosquitoes use to search out their hosts.

Most mosquitoes have a life cycle of about 2 weeks. Hardy females lay about 200 eggs every 10 days. Fortunately, less than 5 percent of the eggs become mature adults, and each fall the initial frost kills most of the adult mosquitoes. Some mosquito eggs, however, may survive for years to decades, hatching when the right combination of warm weather and moisture occurs.

Only female mosquitoes bite people, and they do so only to obtain the blood they need to reproduce. Mosquitoes can fly with a blood meal two to three times their body weight. Some bite only during daylight; others bite only at dusk or at night (Conniff 1977). None, however, like hot afternoons; in fact under those conditions they can die of dehydration.

When biting a victim, a mosquito immediately injects an enzyme, apyrase, that acts on the platelets to assure the continuing flow of blood. The victim's immune system responds by releasing histamines and other substances into the tissue around the bite, causing the blood vessels to dilate and produce swelling and itching.

Mosquitoes appear to be especially attracted to certain odors and gases. One of these is carbon dioxide, which humans exhale with every breath. Some mosquitoes also are attracted by lactic acid, a common by-product of muscle contractions and accompanying perspiration. Mosquitoes also appear to prefer dark colors.

Impacts

Mosquitoes are transmitters of diverse agents of disease. *Anopheles quadrimaculatus,* which breeds in swamps, was the principal vector of malaria in the southeastern United States; *Aedes aegypti,* which breeds predominantly in artificial containers (such as cans, bottles, and old tires), is the urban vector for yellow fever and is also thought to transmit dengue fever, a debilitating viral disease common in parts of Asia, West Africa, and the Americas. Because of increasing concern about AIDS, inquiries have been made about the possible transmission of this infection by mosquitoes (Siemens, 1987). There is strong evidence that the AIDS virus (HIV) cannot survive in mosquitoes. Although it could exist as a contaminant on its mouth parts, the mosquito's mouth is too small to contain sufficient virus particles to provide any likelihood of transmission. In essence, the possibility that mosquitoes transmit the AIDS virus is vanishingly remote.

Control

Control of mosquitoes and mosquito-transmitted infections involves two basic steps: (1) reducing the mosquito population by eliminating their breeding habitats—draining land areas in the case of *Anopheles quadrimaculatus,* or applying insecticides or other agents to kill the adult mosquitoes or their larvae; and (2) preventing mosquitoes from biting people and providing medical treatment to people who have been, or are subject to being, infected. This last step, however, is only ameliorative; it is not possible to attain a sufficient level of medical treatment to influence the transmission of a mosquitoborne disease. Mosquito control is complex because of the large number of species involved and their widely different breeding places, biting habits, flight ranges, and relationship to disease. Shoreline towns may be troubled by salt-marsh mosquitoes, inland towns by freshwater ones.

Agencies planning any type of control program would be wise to hire an entomologist to identify exactly which mosquitoes are the problem and to give advice on the most effective control measures.

Reducing the Population

Whereas earlier programs to kill mosquitoes provided temporary relief at best, the discovery and exploitation of *Bacillus thuringiensis israeliensis* (BTI), a natural enemy of mosquito larvae, have changed this situation dramatically. This bacterium appears to kill only mosquito and black fly larvae; it has shown no toxicity to humans or other nontarget organisms. So far no mosquito larvae have developed resistance to this agent. As a result, BTI is being widely used as a larvicide throughout the world for the control of mosquitoes and is proving spectacularly successful. Other approaches still in use include eliminating breeding zones by digging drainage canals, preventing construction and other practices that lead to the creation of stagnant water, changing the salinity of existing waters, and raising and lowering the water level in lakes, such as those created by dams, to disrupt the life cycle of the mosquito.

Insecticides continue to be widely used to control adult mosquitoes. In the past, the most commonly used insecticide was dichlorodiphenyltrichloroethane (DDT). Because of environmental concerns, its use was banned in the United States in 1972, and certain other organochlorine compounds (such as aldrin and dieldrin) were subsequently banned. The use of DDT has also been banned in Europe and many other parts of the world. Malathion is now the principal insecticide being used. Since *Anopheles* mosquitoes typically bite people at night and then land on the wall to rest, a successful strategy is to apply the insecticide to the inside walls of a house so the mosquitoes will contact it and be killed. Before the development of BTI, DDT was also applied to water areas to kill mosquito larvae. Another larvicide in use today is Abate.

Prevention of Biting

Besides staying indoors except on breezy days or on hot afternoons, people can prevent or at least reduce mosquito bites by placing screens on doors, windows, and porches; by using protective clothing and mosquito netting; and by applying mosquito repellents to the skin.

There is a variety of repellents available commercially (Consumer Reports, 1987). All contain chemicals such as diethyltoluamide (DEET). In deciding which to use, people should try several to determine which is most effective against mosquitoes and most compatible with their skin. Because DEET is harmful to children, only products containing less than 35 percent DEET should be used. Higher concentrations can also damage plastics, such as eyeglasses, and some synthetic fibers. To counteract the attractive odor of perspiration, some people recommend the consumption of vitamin B-1, which will cause perspiration to smell like garlic, an odor that some mosquitoes dislike (Conniff, 1977).

Medical Treatment

Treating people who have been bitten by mosquitoes may range from applying rubbing alcohol on the resulting welt to the administration of drugs, such as chloroquine in the case of malaria. The malaria parasite in Africa has developed resistance to this drug, so it is no longer an effective treatment there. However, chloroquine continues to be effective in South America. Although a vaccine has been developed to prevent yellow fever, efforts to develop one for malaria have not yet been successful (Hoffman et al., 1991).

Flies

Among the members of the fly family, three have been selected for discussion here. One is the housefly (*Musca domestica*), which is present in many of the more temperate parts of the world and is a potential carrier of the agents for numerous diseases. The other two are the screwworm fly (*Cochliomyia hominivorax*), because of its potentially devastating impact on livestock; and the Mediterranean fruitfly (*Ceretitis capitata*), because of its potentially destructive effects on citrus and other fruit.

The Housefly

CHARACTERISTICS

The housefly is gray and about ¼ inch long. It breeds in a variety of decaying animal and vegetable matter, and its larval stage is the maggot. In rural areas, horse, pig, cow, or chicken manure frequently serves as a breeding habitat; human excreta can also be involved where proper disposal methods are not observed.

The housefly's larval stage lasts 4–8 days, the pupal stage 3–6 days. In warm weather, the average time from the laying of eggs to the emergence of the adult is 10–16 days. Flies live 2–8 weeks in midsummer. In cooler weather they may live up to 10 weeks. Although flies have been reported to travel several miles in one day, most flies present in an area have probably originated nearby.

IMPACTS

Although their role in transmitting disease is difficult to document, houseflies pick up and carry a wide range of pathogens (including viruses, bacteria, protozoa, and eggs and cysts of worms), both externally (on their mouth parts, body and leg hairs, and the sticky pads of their feet) and internally (in their intestinal tract). As a rule, however, pathogens picked up by the larvae are not transmitted to the adult fly, and most pathogens picked up by adult flies do not multiply in them. The germs on the surface of a fly often survive only a few hours, especially if exposed to the sun. In contrast, pathogens can live in the intestinal tract and be transmitted to humans when the fly vomits or defecates (Keiding, 1976). In order to eat, the housefly regurgitates a fluid that dissolves its food. Part of this effluent may remain behind on the food when the fly departs and may contain pathogenic organisms. Specific diseases in which houseflies may play a role include typhoid, dysentery, diarrhea, cholera, yaws, and trachoma.

The Screwworm Fly

CHARACTERISTICS

The adult screwworm fly has a metallic blue body and three black stripes on its back between its wings, and is about twice as large as the housefly. In contrast to the housefly, the screwworm fly lays its eggs in fresh wounds of warm-blooded animals. Any accidental or surgical wound, a fresh brand mark, or the navel of a newborn animal can serve as the site for initial invasion by screwworm maggots. In warm areas populated by screwworm flies, few newborn calves, lambs, kids, pigs, or the young of the larger game species escape attack.

The maggots hatch in 12–24 hours and begin feeding on the flesh head-down, soon invading the sound tissue. The feeding larvae cause a straw-colored and often bloody discharge that attracts more flies, resulting in multiple infestations by hundreds to thousands of maggots of all sizes. Death is inevitable in the case of an intense infestation unless the animal is found and treated (Knipling, 1960).

The maggots become full grown in about 5 days. They then drop out of the wound, burrow into the ground, and change to the pupal or resting stage. The adult flies emerge from the pupal case after about 8 days during warm weather, live for 2–3 weeks, and range for many miles (Knipling, 1960).

IMPACTS

Early in the twentieth century, screwworm flies were present in southern Texas and northern Mexico and annually migrated northward into Louisiana and Arkansas. In 1933 screwworm flies appeared in Georgia, presumably introduced through shipment of infested cattle from the Southwest. During that summer screwworm flies spread southward into Florida, where they were a problem in the 1930s and early 1940s. Subsequent outbreaks occurred in the United States in the late 1950s, in 1972–1976, and again in 1978 (Richardson, Ellison, and Averhoff, 1982).

Screwworm flies can have devastating effects on livestock growers. Losses from screwworm infestations along the Atlantic seaboard in 1958 were estimated at $20 million (Richardson, Ellison, and Averhoff, 1982). Today losses from a major outbreak would be many times that amount. For this reason, ranchers in states such as Texas and Florida gladly pay a tax per head of cattle to finance control programs. The screwworm fly continues to be a problem in Central and South America, and recently, a related species has appeared in Africa. The 2-year eradication program developed for use there in the early 1990s is estimated to have cost $117 million (Palca, 1990).

The Mediterranean Fruitfly

CHARACTERISTICS

The Mediterranean fruitfly, also known as the Medfly, is slightly smaller than the common housefly, has yellowish-orange spots on its

wings, and thrives in a warm climate. Scientists believe that it originated in West Africa. By 1850 it had spread throughout the Mediterranean region; it was found in Australia in the late 1800s, and in Brazil
and Hawaii in the early 1900s. In 1929 it was discovered in Florida
(World Book Encyclopedia, 1990).

A Medfly typically lays her eggs in a ripe, preferably acidic, fruit
while it is still on the tree. Preferred targets are oranges, grapefruit,
peaches, nectarines, plums, apples, and quinces. The Medfly drills
tiny holes in the skin or rind and lays 2–6 eggs in each hole. The eggs
hatch in 2–20 days into larvae, which eat their way through the fruit,
causing it to drop to the ground. The larvae later burrow into the
ground, where they pupate. Adult flies emerge after some 10–50 days.

IMPACTS

Although quarantines of fruit and other measures have brought the
Medfly under control, infestations recurred in Florida and Texas between 1930 and 1979, and again in 1984, 1985, and 1987. The Medfly
also appeared in California in 1975, 1980, 1987, and 1990. Because the
export of fruit is prohibited from any areas where the Medfly has been
detected, the economic impact is tremendous.

Control

Several approaches can be used to control flies. The specific technique
depends on the habits of the given species.

SANITATION

Although installing screens in buildings helps reduce contact between
houseflies and people, it does nothing to reduce the fly population.
This requires other approaches, one of the most important of which
is a good sanitation program. Keeping garbage and excreta covered
and disposing of them promptly and properly will eliminate major
breeding grounds for houseflies. Prompt disposal of garbage, especially decaying fruit, and prompt removal and disposal of infested fruit
that has fallen from trees have proved effective in controlling the
Mediterranean fruitfly in countries such as Israel and Italy. These
measures, however, have essentially no effect on the screwworm fly.

One approach for its control is to restrict the breeding of cattle so that births occur only during the winter months, when the screwworm fly population is at a minimum.

INSECTICIDES

Chemical insecticides are widely used for controlling flies. They can be wiped or sprayed on indoor surfaces to kill houseflies, or tapes impregnated with insecticides can be hung from the ceiling. Care must be taken, however, to avoid contamination of foodstuffs. Outdoor control measures include the application of larvicides to breeding areas and the use of bait stations and sprays.

Initially the principal insecticides used for killing adult flies were the organochlorine compounds, such as DDT, dieldrin, and chlordane. All of these except DDT were found to be extremely toxic to humans. They also proved to be persistent, remaining in the environment for long periods. In addition, because of its persistence and the fact it was bioaccumulated in the environment, DDT was found to have adverse effects on birds (through decalcification of their eggshells), fish, and bats. Recently there has been a shift to the far less persistent organophosphorus compounds (such as malathion, used to control the screwworm fly and Mediterranean fruitfly), the carbamates (such as Sevin), and the pyrethroids (such as permethrin).

Since flies, even more than mosquitoes, have become resistant to virtually all insecticides, insecticides cannot and should not be used as the sole means of control.

RADIATION STERILIZATION

Radiation sterilization was developed in the late 1950s and led to the eradication of the screwworm fly in the United States. Although the results of this effort proved to be temporary, the technique remains a very effective method for the control of this insect. It consists in artificially breeding and growing millions of adult males, sterilizing them with radiation, and then releasing them into an area, so that eggs of the indigenous female flies with which they mate do not hatch. The technique benefits from the fact that insects generally mate only once, but it is applicable only where the density of the fly population is low, so that sufficient numbers of sterile males can be released to have an impact. Radiation sterilization is now being used in Mexico, Belize, and Guatemala against the screwworm fly and is being considered for use against the Mediterranean fruitfly in Egypt and the screwworm fly in Libya (Palca, 1990).

Implications of Insecticide Use

The use of insecticides for controlling insect pests, especially in agriculture, dates at least to 1690, when, for example, tobacco was used in France to combat lace bugs that were infesting pear trees. Pyrethrum, a compound obtained from the chrysanthemum family, was used in 1800 to kill fleas. Rotenone, which can be extracted from various plants, was used in 1848 to control leaf-eating caterpillars; and "Paris green" (copper acetoarsenite) was used against the Colorado potato beetle in the late 1860s. Today insecticides are being widely used for the control of a host of insects. In many cases, though, their application and use have resulted in harm to people and to the environment.

The most widely known and used modern insecticide is DDT. This material was first synthesized in 1874, but its insecticide properties were not discovered until 1939. Beginning in 1943, the U.S. Army used it on a limited basis to control fleas during a typhus epidemic in Naples, Italy. In 1960 the World Health Organization introduced its use worldwide.

The success of DDT prompted the development and introduction of a host of similar chemical derivatives, including chlordane, heptachlor, aldrin, dieldrin, toxaphene, and endrin. Use of these materials has led to contamination of human food and animal feed; contamination of clothing, with subsequent absorption of the chemicals into the body; harmful effects on birds (for example, the pelican) through bioaccumulation in the environment; and contamination of large groundwater and surface water supplies as a result of seepage and runoff from agricultural lands. In 1984 an accident at an insecticide manufacturing plant in Bhopal, India, led to the release of large amounts of a pesticide into the environment and killed more than 2,000 people.

Exacerbating these problems, insects have developed resistance to these chemicals, and in response farmers have increased the amounts they use. From 1970 to 1980, for example, the number of arthropod species resistant to pesticides increased from an estimated 200 to almost 450. Thirty-six countries report that 25 species of beetles, caterpillars, mites, and other insects that attack cotton plants are now resistant to pesticides. And 84 countries report that the malaria-carrying *Anopheles* mosquito is resistant to one or more of the major insecticide groups (Georghiuo, 1985). Scientists do not know how to monitor or control this increase in insect resistance (Gianessi, 1987). For these and other reasons, the trend in many parts of the world is to use an integrated approach to the management of insects.

Integrated Pest Management

The integrated approach to pest control is based on acquiring complete information about a given insect (including its physiology, predators, and life cycle), the technical measures available, and the political, industrial, and environmental factors involved, and then using a combination of strategies. Planning of the control program occurs at the local level with full input from the community. If the problem is agricultural, for example, strategies may include rotating crops to interrupt the cycle of specific pests, interspersing one crop with another to confuse insects, carefully timing control efforts (that is, applying pesticides only when insects appear and using them only in carefully controlled amounts), introducing natural predators to combat specific pests, and applying an insecticide developed specifically for a given pest. Although the integrated approach requires time, especially at the planning stage, once launched it tends to be self-perpetuating.

The General Outlook

With the recognition that widespread use of pesticides can severely affect human health and the environment, efforts have increased to develop new procedures for controlling insects and rodents. One novel approach involves the use of giant vacuum cleaners in the field to remove insects from strawberry plants (Driscoll Strawberry Associates, 1989). A more promising trend is to seek out natural predators for specific insects. In fact this approach is far from new: in ancient China, predatory ants were released on trees to protect them from destructive pests (Best, 1989). More recently a tiny green lacewing, a natural predator that feasts on insects, has been used successfully to protect pecan trees in New Mexico; ants have been used in Cuba to protect banana trees from insect pests; and the bacterium BTI is being used worldwide to kill mosquito and black fly larvae.

A large-scale search for natural insecticides will require increased entomological research (Holden, 1989). Of the estimated 10 million insect species in the world today, only 750,000 have been identified. Once insects are identified, their life cycles and habits must be studied as well as any compounds they secrete that might be used to control other insects. Some millipedes, for example, have been found to emit a chemical related to Quaalude that can paralyze a spider for hours; centipede mothers spread a substance on their eggs that acts as a fungicide; and some beetles contain steroids that may lower the fecundity of predators. The quest for natural insecticides, however, must take into account that many products occurring in nature are extremely toxic and may simply create new and different problems. Before widespread use, they must be evaluated as carefully as artificially produced pesticides.

REFERENCES

American Public Health Association. 1990. "Tropical Diseases Affect One-Tenth the World's Population." *Nation's Health* 20, no. 7 (July) 8–9.
Best, Cheryl. 1989. "Natural Pest Controls." *Garbage* 1, no. 1 (September/October), 40–46.
Canby, Thomas Y. 1977. "The Rat—Lapdog of the Devil." *National Geographic* 152, no. 1 (July), 60–87.
Conniff, Richard. 1977. "The Malevolent Mosquito." *Reader's Digest* 111, no. 664 (August), 153–157.
Consumer Reports. 1987. "Insect Repellants." *Consumer Reports* 52, no. 7 (July), 423–426.
Driscoll Strawberry Associates. 1989. "Giant 'Vacuum Cleaner' Solving Pest Problem for Leading California Strawberry Producer." News release. Watsonville, Calif.
Duplaix, Nicole. 1988. "Fleas, the Lethal Leapers." *National Geographic* 173, no. 5 (May), 672–694.
Fischer, Karl C. 1969. *Environment and Health,* Chap. 6. Loma Linda, Calif.: Loma Linda University Printing Service.
Georghiuo, G. P. 1985. "Pesticide Resistance Management." *NewsReport* (National Research Council) 35, no. 2 (February), 28–29.

Gianessi, L. P. 1987. "Lack of Data Stymies Informed Decisions on Agricultural Pesticides." *Resources,* no. 89 (Fall), 1–4.

Guest, Charles. 1984. "The Pied Piper of Hamelin." *Lancet,* 22/29 December, pp. 1454–1455.

Hoffman, Stephen L., Victor Nussenzweig, Jerald C. Sadoff, and Ruth S. Nussenzweig. 1991. "Progress toward Malaria Preerythrocytic Vaccine." *Science* 252, no. 5005 (26 April), 520–521.

Holden, Constance. 1989. "Entomologists Wane as Insects Wax." *Science* 246, no. 4931 (10 November), 754–756.

Keiding, J. 1976. *The House-Fly—Biology and Control,* Report WHO/VBC/76.650. Geneva: World Health Organization.

Knipling, Edward F. 1960. "The Eradication of the Screw-Worm Fly." *Scientific* American 203, no. 4 (October), 54–61.

Lore, Richard, and Kevin Flannelly. 1977. "Rat Societies." *Scientific American* 236, no. 5, (May), 106–116.

Palca, Joseph. 1990. "Libya Gets Unwelcome Visitor from the West." *Science* 249, no. 4965 (13 July), 117–118.

Richardson, R. H., J. R. Ellison, and W. W. Averhoff. 1982. "Autocidal Control of Screwworms in North America." Science 215, no. 4531 (22 January), 361–370.

Siemens, D. F., Jr. 1987. "AIDS Transmission and Insects." Letter to the editor. *Science* 238, no. 4824 (9 October), 143.

Spielman, Andrew. 1991. Private communication to author. Harvard University, School of Public Health.

Weinstein, Jack S. 1990. *Lyme Disease.* New York: American Council of Science and Health.

World Book Encyclopedia. 1990. 13th ed. Chicago: World Book.

8

Injury Control

After heart disease, cancer, and stroke, accidents are the leading cause of death in the United States. They account for almost 100,000 deaths and some 8–10 million disabling injuries each year (National Safety Council, 1990). About 50,000 people are killed in vehicular accidents and about the same number altogether in community and recreational activities, fires, drownings, and work-related accidents. Many environmental and public health officials regard accidental deaths and injuries as the most underrecognized public health problem.

Accidents are the leading cause of death for both sexes until about age 40. Accidents account for almost 40 percent of the deaths of 1-to-4-year-olds and for almost 50 percent for ages 5–14 and 15–24. For 15-to-24-year-olds, accidents claim about three times more lives than the next leading cause of death, and motor vehicle accidents account for almost 80 percent of these deaths. More than three out of four accident victims in this age group are males (National Safety Council, 1990). About 20 million 1-to-14-year-olds are injured in accidents each year, and 60 percent of these accidents occur in or near the home (Nelson and Whittenberger, 1977). In the United States, accidents cause almost 300 deaths per day; another 170,000 people are injured seriously enough to require medical attention.

The economic cost of accidents in the United States is estimated at almost $150 billion per year. This includes the associated medical expenses, insurance administration costs, lost wages, and property damage. Not included are the costs of public agencies such as police, courts, and fire departments and indirect losses to employers from employees' off-the-job accidents and subsequent absenteeism. Because accidents predominantly kill people in the younger age groups, assessment of the associated impacts must also include the many years of productivity lost through the unfulfilled lives of its victims (National Safety Council, 1990).

While motor vehicles account for the most accidental deaths in the United States, work-related accidents continue to be important. During 1989 about 1.7 million workers suffered disabling injuries, and more than 10,000 were killed. About 31 percent of these injuries resulted from overexertion; another 24 percent resulted from being struck by or struck against an object. More than one third (37 percent) of the fatalities involved work-related accidents in motor vehicles. Falls were the next-highest contributor (13 percent) (National Safety Council, 1990). Over half of the deaths occurred in the 25-to-44-year-old work group, and 94 percent of those killed were males (CDC, 1989). Annual fatality rates per 100,000 workers were highest for mine and quarry workers, farmers, construction workers, and transportation operatives (Table 8.1). Overall, significant progress is being made in reducing accidental death rates for workers. The death rate in 1989

Table 8.1   Deaths and injuries for various industrial groups, 1989

Group	Number of deaths per year		Number of disabling injuries
	Total	per 100,000	
Mining and quarrying	300	43	30,000
Agriculture[a]	1,300	40	120,000
Construction	2,100	32	190,000
Transportation and public utilities	1,400	24	140,000
Government	1,600	9	240,000
Manufacturing	1,100	6	340,000
Trade	1,100	4	340,000
Services[b]	1,500	4	300,000
All industries	10,400	9	1,700,000

a. Includes forestry and fishing.
b. Includes finance, insurance, and real estate.

was less than half of that in 1960. However, the cost of work-related accidents remains high, an estimated $50 billion in 1989 (National Safety Council, 1990).

This chapter surveys the strategies that can prevent or reduce injuries and deaths from accidents.

The Environmental, Scientific, and Public Health Approach to Injury Control

According to Julian Waller (1989), injury control as a public health endeavor began in Germany in 1780, when Johann Frank urged that injury and its prevention be addressed not only by individuals but also by nationwide public health programs. In the mid-1900s, several state and local health departments in the United States initiated modest data collection efforts and child safety, burn prevention, and other programs. Few of these, however, followed up with evaluations of the programs' effects on behavior, morbidity, or mortality.

In 1942 Hugh De Haven, an engineer at Cornell University, published a paper (De Haven, 1942) that began a conceptual revolution in injury control. By showing how people successfully survived falls of 50–150 feet, in some cases with only minor injury, through proper dispersion of kinetic energy in amounts as great as 200 times the force of gravity, he demonstrated that it is possible to disconnect the linkage between accidents and the resultant injuries. De Haven's studies led to the development and introduction of seat belts and other occupant restraints as an effective method of reducing injuries in automobile accidents (Waller, 1987).

In 1961 J. J. Gibson observed that there are only five agents of all injury events, namely, the five forms of physical energy: kinetic or mechanical energy, chemical energy, thermal energy, electricity, and radiation (Gibson, 1961). Expanding upon this new concept of injury causation, in the early 1960s Dr. William Haddon, then at the New York State Department of Health, launched a movement to base accident and injury prevention programs on sounder scientific and public health concepts. He applied an environmental approach to injury control instead of relying primarily on attempts to change human behavior. With the 1970s came federal programs to deal with threats to health in the environment, but most programs addressing accidental injuries targeted the workplace.

Current efforts combine broadened application of Haddon's concepts and strategies (discussed below) with sophisticated use of behavioral interventions. This approach reflects the growing awareness since the 1970s that injuries cannot be reduced without changes in the attitudes and behaviors of the target population.

Haddon developed a generic approach to the analysis, management, and control of accidents, which he treated as fundamentally a result of the rapid and uncontrolled transfer of energy (Haddon, 1970). This approach can be applied to all types of occupational and environmental hazards, ranging from automobile accidents to oil spills to a major accident in a nuclear power plant.

Accident Phases

To facilitate an analytic approach, Haddon divided accidents into three phases: the pre-event phase (which includes all the factors that determine whether an accident occurs), the event itself, and the post-event phase (which includes everything that determines the consequences of the injuries received). The factors operating in all three phases are the humans involved, the equipment they are using or with which they come into contact, and the environment in which the equipment is being operated. Combining the three accident phases and these three factors yields a nine-cell matrix (Figure 8.1) that public health workers can use to determine where best to apply strategies to prevent or control injuries. Because vehicular accidents account for about half the accidental fatalities in the United States, they are used as examples in the following discussion.

Pre-Event Phase

Factors that should be considered during this phase include:

Humans involved: driver impairment by alcohol or other drugs; the thoroughness of testing procedures for licensure; the degree of enforcement of traffic rules and regulations, including mandatory use of seat belts; and the availability of mass transportation as an alternative to the use of private vehicles

Equipment: the condition of brakes, headlights, and tire treads; the size and visibility of brake lights; the speed the vehicle can attain; and vehicular crash tests

PHASES	FACTORS		
	HUMAN	EQUIPMENT	PHYSICAL AND SOCIOECONOMIC ENVIRONMENT
PRE-EVENT	(1)	(2)	(3)
EVENT	(4)	(5)	(6)
POST-EVENT	(7)	(8)	(9)

Figure 8.1   Matrix for the analysis of accidents

Environment: the presence of barriers and traffic lights to protect
pedestrians; the design, placement, and maintenance of road
signs for ready comprehension; and the design of roads and
bridge abutments

Event Phase

Factors that can reduce the extent of injuries during this phase include:

Humans involved: occupants' use of vehicles equipped with air
bags, proper use of seat belts and child-restraint systems, and
driver abstention from alcohol (because alcohol affects cell mem-
brane permeability, even in low-impact collisions people who
have consumed alcohol are more likely to sustain severe or even
fatal neurological damage)

Equipment: a collapsible steering column, high-penetration-
resistant windshield, interior padding (for example, on the dash-
board), recessed door handles and control knobs, and structural
beams in doors; low bumpers with square fronts to reduce the
likelihood of pelvic and leg fractures in pedestrians who are hit;

and, on trucks, a bar under the rear end to prevent cars from "submarining" beneath them

Environment: breakaway sign posts, open space along the sides of the road, wide multiple lanes, and guard rails to steer vehicles back onto the road

Post-Event Phase

Factors that can reduce or limit the effects of injuries in this phase include:

Humans involved: rapid and appropriate emergency medical care, followed by adequate rehabilitation; properly trained associated rescue personnel; and injury severity scores to help medical personnel evaluate multiple traumas and predict outcomes

Equipment: fireproof gasoline tanks to prevent fires after an accident

Environment: public telephones along the roadway for summoning emergency help, "jaws of life" to extract victims from vehicles, helicopters for rapid transport of victims to medical care facilities, and trauma centers equipped to handle injured victims

Much the same approach can be used to analyze other types of accidents and strategies to prevent or limit associated injuries.

Haddon's 10 Strategies

Expanding on his generic approach, Haddon identified 10 strategies that could reduce the damage from all kinds of hazards (Haddon, 1980):

Strategy 1: Prevent the marshalling of the form of energy that leads to the accident. Specific examples include installing barriers to prevent babies from crawling on top of cabinets or into windows from which they can fall, limiting the height of all buildings to one story, forbidding the manufacture of explosives and of consumer products that are known to be harmful to individuals or the environment, and discontinuing the construction and operation of nuclear power plants. A still more extreme example would include preventing the movement of vehicles.

Strategy 2: Reduce the amount of energy that can be marshalled or brought into being. Examples include restricting the speeds that transportation vehicles can attain, limiting the power level of nuclear plants so as to restrict the quantities of radionuclides available for release in case of a major accident, limiting the height of diving boards above swimming pools, reducing the amounts and concentrations of chemical reagents that can be used in high school laboratory experiments, administering baby (small) aspirin instead of adult aspirin to children, and limiting the amount of explosives that can be contained in firecrackers.

Strategy 3: Prevent the release of the energy from existing sources. The major avenue is behavioral intervention. This strategy would include encouraging people to obey traffic laws, prohibiting the sale of matches, requiring that household cleansers and other toxic agents be sold only in containers with childproof caps, requiring window washers to wear safety belts, strengthening mine roofs by bolting and timbering, making certain that scaffolding is so strong and firmly affixed that it cannot fall, and diluting combustibles and other energy sources so that they are no longer capable of releasing their energy.

Strategy 4: Modify the rate or spatial distribution of the release of energy from its source. Examples include using seat belts and air bags to protect passengers in motor vehicles, reducing the slope of ski trails for beginners, and using parachutes in falls through the air.

Strategy 5: Separate in space or time the energy being released and the people to be protected. Examples include eliminating or separating vehicles and their pathways from areas commonly used by children and adults, placing electric power lines on tall poles out of the reach of people, evacuating population groups following the accidental release of large quantities of toxic chemicals into the environment, banning vehicles carrying explosives from tunnels and congested urban areas, erecting vehicular barriers at railroad crossings, and using rods to route the energy in lightning past susceptible people and structures (Waller, 1987).

Strategy 6: Install a barrier between the energy being released and the people to be protected. Examples include safety shoes, safety glasses, protective helmets, lead aprons for x-ray technicians, guards on electric table saws, insulation on electric wiring, thermal shields, and containments around nuclear power reactors.

Strategy 7: Modify the surface, subsurface, or basic structure of various everyday objects (for example, by eliminating, rounding, or softening corners, edges, and points with which people can come into contact) so as to reduce the injuries caused by sudden contact. Although this strategy is now increasingly reflected in automobile design, it has been overlooked for years in the designs of buildings and a host of consumer products. Much could be done in designing nurseries, hospitals, and nursing homes to reduce many of the injuries that occur daily in such facilities. Other examples of this strategy include installing breakaway poles along the sides of roads and making lollipop sticks out of cardboard.

Strategy 8: Strengthen the structure, living or nonliving, to limit the damage that it might otherwise receive as a result of the energy transfer. Examples include more-stringent design codes for buildings to withstand earthquakes, hurricanes, and fires, and for motor vehicles to withstand collisions. In public health, this strategy would include training athletes to increase muscle mass, preventing or treating osteoporosis, and using vaccines, such as those for polio, yellow fever, and smallpox, to reduce the impact of these infectious diseases.

Strategy 9: If the strategies above have not been used or have been used ineffectively, and if an accident has occurred and damage has resulted, assess the damage and take steps as quickly as possible to stop or contain it. Examples include providing prompt and effective emergency medical care to the injured, giving stable iodine to people potentially exposed to radioiodine from accidental releases from nuclear power plants, using fire suppression systems (for example, water sprinklers) in buildings, and providing drinking water, excreta disposal, and shelter to victims of earthquakes and floods.

Strategy 10: Stabilize, repair, and rehabilitate the structures that have been damaged. Examples include cosmetic surgery following trauma, physical therapy for amputees and others with disabling injuries, repairing damaged buildings, reconstructing roads, and replanting agricultural crops.

Vehicular Accidents

Each year in the United States vehicular accidents cause approximately 50,000 deaths; they are the leading cause of death up through

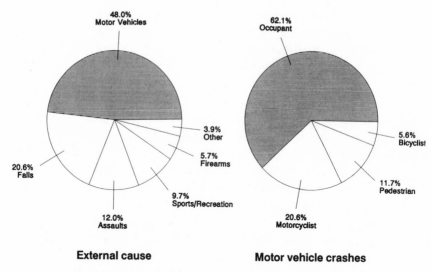

48.0%
Motor Vehicles

62.1%
Occupant

3.9%
Other

5.7%
Firearms

9.7%
Sports/Recreation

20.6%
Falls

12.0%
Assaults

5.6%
Bicyclist

11.7%
Pedestrian

20.6%
Motorcyclist

External cause   **Motor vehicle crashes**

Figure 8.2   Distribution of brain injuries by external cause and from motor
vehicle crashes, San Diego County, California, 1981

age 40. They also account for 4–5 million injuries, including almost half of all cases involving brain damage (Figure 8.2) and more than half of all traumatic spinal cord injuries (Insurance Institute for Highway Safety, 1989). Almost 100,000 hospital personnel and over 10 percent of all hospital beds are devoted to patients injured in vehicular accidents. The associated annual economic costs of these accidents are estimated to exceed $70 billion (National Safety Council, 1990). Because so many of the victims are younger people, the loss in years of life is also very high. Preventing or reducing the problem has political, social, behavioral, and economic aspects and requires a multifaceted approach. The subjects that must be addressed include:

Human-factors engineering: Human-factors engineering, or ergonomics, should play a large role in vehicle design, to eliminate the possibility of the driver's mistaking the controls (such as pushing on the gas pedal instead of the brake), to ensure that all controls are within easy reach, and to provide a clear and unobstructed view of the road and pedestrians. Ergonomics can also address the problem of drivers who consume alcohol. Since it is often difficult to get such drivers to change their behavior through public education campaigns alone, vehicles could be equipped with a system of pushbuttons requiring the driver to enter a specific sequence of numbers before the vehicle can be started.

Protection of occupants: Vehicles must be designed so that occupants are protected in the event of a crash. In addition to the items mentioned above, cars should have head restraints that protect against whiplash and doors that will remain closed so that people are not thrown outside.

Control of the operating environment: The carnage of vehicular accidents can be significantly reduced through improved highway design that better accommodates driver error. So that cars accidentally leaving the road can come to a safe stop, highways bordered by open fields should not have guard rails. Trees that are too close to roadways should be removed. On city streets, signs and pedestrian walkways should be clearly lit. Finally, controlled access should be provided whenever possible on both rural and urban roads.

Prompt emergency medical care and rehabilitation: Speed of response and level and quality of medical care are important elements in helping people injured in accidents. Wartime experience has demonstrated conclusively that many of even the most seriously injured people can be saved if they receive prompt emergency medical care and adequate subsequent rehabilitation. With the increasing use of helicopters and emergency medical teams, the prospects for the survival of victims of highway or traffic accidents are improving (Wynn, 1990).

Accidents Involving Children

In the developed countries, accidents contribute to far more injuries and deaths among children than do communicable diseases. In the United States accidents account for 44 percent of the deaths among 1-to-14-year-olds (National Safety Council, 1990). Given these statistics, it seems strange that health agencies spend millions of dollars annually on programs to combat leukemia and muscular dystrophy but very little on the prevention and control of accidental injuries and deaths. One problem is a general lack of data on which to base planning efforts. Massachusetts is an exception. Extensive studies there

have shown that every year 1 of every 5 children is injured and requires treatment in a hospital, 1 of every 50 teenagers is injured in
automobile accidents, 1 of every 12 children under age 5 requires
hospital treatment for falls, 29 percent of all injuries to teenagers occur
in the workplace, and sports deaths (which gain much publicity when
they occur) are minimal in comparison with other causes of death
among young people (Gallagher et al., 1984).

But the main problem thwarting large-scale programs to reduce
deaths and injuries, at least among small children, is that control of
accidents is heavily dependent on parents' awareness of potential hazards and their behavior as a result. With enough public education,
however, parents could use many of the strategies described above.
Specifically, they could provide child-resistant cabinet doors for the
storage of household cleansers and other toxic agents; fit stairs with
handrails and padding; fence play yards; cover the ground beneath
swings, slides, and other playground equipment with soft earth (versus clay or asphalt); and closely supervise young children when they
are outdoors.

Legislated codes and standards can also play an important role in
reducing childhood injuries. Examples include the requirements that
all toxic materials be sold in containers with childproof caps; that
hot-water heaters have temperature limits to prevent scalds and
burns; that barriers be installed on upstairs windows of buildings; that
fences be erected around swimming pools; that playground equipment
be designed to prevent entrapment, falls, and contact with protruding
parts; that electrical outlets near the floor be covered; that paint used
on indoor walls, furniture, and equipment for children be lead-free;
and that control knobs on stoves be located out of children's reach.

Fires

Although the United States has more buildings with smoke alarms
and sprinklers and more fire fighters than any other country, data
reported by the Federal Emergency Management Agency (FEMA)
show that the death rate from fires is 1.5 to 3 times that in most other
developed countries (1990). In 1989 more than 4,000 people in the
United States died in fires (National Safety Council, 1990). One of the
reasons for this high death rate is that many smoke detectors are
incorrectly located or installed or are nonoperational because of dead

or missing batteries. As is the case for accidents involving motor vehicles and children, data on causes, places of occurrence, and effects provide useful information on possible strategies to prevent or reduce injuries and deaths from fires. For example:

Residential fires account for about 21 percent of those reported, but for 75 percent of the deaths, 67 percent of the injuries, and almost half of all property loss (FEMA, 1990).

In residences the leading cause of fires (22 percent) is a defective local heating system, often installed to supplement or replace a central heating system. These supplementary systems include both fixed units such as wood-burning stoves, stationary electric heaters, and fireplaces, and portable units such as kerosene, electric, and gas space heaters. The increased use of both fixed and portable supplementary heating devices has been paralleled by a substantial increase in fires (FEMA, 1990). The leading cause of deaths in residential fires is cigarette smoking (29 percent). For all types of fires, the leading cause of injuries (19 percent) and economic loss (18 percent) is arson (National Safety Council, 1990).

The highest death rates from fires occur in the poorest areas, primarily in the southeastern and south-central states; and of the major cities, the newer ones in the West have the lowest death rates (FEMA, 1984).

Death rates from fires in rural areas are more than twice as high as those in urban areas (Gomberg and Clark, 1982).

Seventy percent of men killed in fires were drunk at the time (Berl and Halpin, 1979).

These data indicate that the three major risk factors associated with deaths from fires are poverty, cigarettes, and alcohol.

As with most environmental and public health problems, the control of deaths and injuries from fires requires a systems approach. Increased fire-fighting capabilities, stricter enforcement of building and housing codes, and intensified pursuit of arsonists are all helpful, but these approaches alone will not eliminate fires or fatalities from them. These activities must be supplemented by the installation and continued maintenance of smoke detectors and sprinkler systems in buildings; increased attention to the design, installation, operation, and maintenance of heating systems, particularly portable units; requirements that sleeping garments, especially those worn by children, be fire-resistant; and the requirement that bedding and upholstered furniture be not only fire-resistant but also incapable of releasing toxic gases when exposed to heat and flame. Few people are burned to death in fires; most die from inhaling smoke and poisonous gases. For example, the high death toll of 43 in a fire in a discothèque in Spain in January 1990 did not stem from the fire itself, which was minor. The deaths occurred when people inhaled hydrocyanic acid, produced by combustion of acrylic fibers used in interior decorations. This compound was taken up and distributed through the ventilation system.

The General Outlook

In the 1980s the number of accidental deaths in the United States declined more than during any other decade on record, from 105,312 in 1979 to 95,600 in 1989, a decrease of 10 percent. The rate at which people died in accidents also decreased over the decade, from 46.9 to 38.1 per 100,000 people per year, a decrease of 19 percent. Motor vehicle deaths dropped by 20 percent, work-related accidents by 29 percent, and home accidents by 16 percent (National Safety Council, 1990).

Factors that are thought to have helped reduce vehicular deaths include state seat belt laws and the accompanying increase in seat belt use, state minimum drinking-age laws, and anti–drinking and driving programs. One attempt to change the behavior of drivers appears to be having an unusual impact and offers hope for continued improvements in the future. This is the Harvard School of Public Health program, launched in 1987, to promote the concept of the "Designated Driver." The School has persuaded television and motion picture producers to give broad coverage to the slogan "The Designated Driver is the Life of the Party"; it has also promoted the concept through spot announcements, posters, and practical manuals for use by communities wishing to implement such a program. There are probably several reasons for the success of the program: the concept is simple; encouraging the use of a designated driver moves away from the overused, negative dictum "Don't drink and drive"; and the selection of the designated driver is a process that reinforces growing social consciousness about the unacceptability of driving after drinking (Winsten, 1990).

In contrast, the number of deaths in the United States from accidents in homes remained unchanged during the 1980s. In 1989, for example, they caused 22,500 deaths and 3,400,000 disabling injuries. About 90,000 of these injuries resulted in some permanent impairment. Although fatalities from poison gas, fires, and falls decreased, these gains were offset by increases in deaths from suffocation and poisoning by solids and liquids. In the decade 1979–1989 deaths from suffocation increased by over 30 percent; deaths from poisoning by solids and liquids nearly doubled (from 2,500 to 4,700). In fact, after falls, poisoning is now the second leading cause of deaths in homes. This increase is entirely due to drug-related deaths, particularly among 25-to-40-year-olds. This age group experienced a 50 percent increase in accidental home deaths in the 1980s (National Safety Council, 1990).

Although the death rate from home accidents for people aged 65 and older decreased by 11 percent in 1979–1989, there was such an increase in the population in this age group that the total number of deaths increased. For people up through age 79, motor-vehicle accidents are the most common type of fatal accident, with falls second. For people 80 and older, falls are the leading cause of death.

Although it is widely accepted that the home and community environment is a major source of accidental deaths and injuries, far too often the impacts of this environment on behavioral patterns of people are overlooked. Consider the fact that some 50,000 people in the United States die each year as a result of suicides and homicides. Public health officials must consider the environment as a totality. Promotion of a healthful environment must include encouraging strong family ties as well as providing ample opportunities, especially to young people, for employment and education.

REFERENCES

Berl, Walter G., and Byron M. Halpin. 1979. "Human Fatalities from Unwanted Fires." *Fire Journal* 73, no. 5 (September), 105–115 and 123.
CDC. 1989. *National Traumatic Occupational Fatalities: 1980–1985*. Cincinnati: National Institute for Occupational Safety and Health, U.S. Department of Health and Human Services.

De Haven, H. 1942. "Mechanical Analysis of Survival in Falls from Heights of Fifty to One Hundred and Fifty Feet." *War Medicine* 2, pp. 586–596.

FEMA. 1984. *Fire in the United States: 1981.* 4th ed. Washington, D.C.

——— 1990. *Fire in the United States: 1983–1987 and Highlights for 1988.* 7th ed. Washington, D.C.

Gallagher, S. S.; K. Finison; B. Guyer; and S. Goodenough. 1984. "The Incidence of Injuries among 87,000 Massachusetts Children and Adolescents: Results of the 1980–81 Statewide Childhood Injury Prevention Program Surveillance System." *American Journal of Public Health* 74, no. 12 (December), 1340–47.

Gibson, J. J., 1961. "Contribution of Experimental Psychology to the Formulation of the Problem of Safety: A Brief for Basic Research." In *Behavioral Approaches to Accident Research*. New York: Association for the Aid of Crippled Children.

Gomberg, A., and L. P. Clark. 1982. *Rural and Non-Rural Civilian Fire Fatalities in Twelve States*. Report of the Federal Emergency Management Agency. Washington, D.C.

Haddon, William, Jr. 1970. "On the Escape of Tigers: An Ecologic Note." *American Journal of Public Health* 60, no. 12, pp. 2229–34.

——— 1980. "The Basic Strategies for Reducing Damage from Hazards of All Kinds." *Hazard Prevention*, September/October, pp. 8–12.

Insurance Institute for Highway Safety. 1989. *Twenty Years of Accomplishment by the Insurance Institute for Highway Safety*. Arlington, Va.

National Safety Council. 1990. *Accident Facts, 1990 Edition*. Chicago.

Nelson, Norton, and James W. Whittenberger. 1977. *Human Health and the Environment: Some Research Needs*. DHEW Publication NIH 77-1277. Washington, D.C.: U.S. Government Printing Office.

Waller, Julian A. 1987. "Injury: Conceptual Shifts and Preventive Implications." *Annual Review of Public Health* 8, 21–49.

——— 1989. "Injury Control in Perspective." Editorial. *American Journal of Public Health* 79, no. 3 (March), 272–273.

Winsten, Jay. 1990. "The Designated Driver Campaign." Status Report, Harvard Alcohol Project, School of Public Health, Harvard University.

Wynn, Jane. 1990. "Emergency Air Transport: Programs, Patient Care, Payment, and Standards." *Standardization News* 18, no. 8 (August), 32–34.

9

Electromagnetic Radiation

All human beings are constantly exposed to natural radiation, artificial radiation, or both. Radiation is thus an ideal form of energy with which to demonstrate the principles used by environmental health professionals to monitor, evaluate, and control physical factors in the occupational and ambient environments. This chapter describes the principal characteristics and sources of electromagnetic radiation, how it interacts with people, its associated biological effects, and methods for monitoring and controlling it.

Electromagnetic radiation is propagated through space in the form of packets of energy called photons. All photons travel at the speed of light (3×10^{10} cm per second), and each has an associated frequency and wavelength. The energy of a photon is directly proportional to its frequency and is expressed in terms of electron volts (eV)—the energy that an electron would acquire in being accelerated across an electrical potential difference of one volt. An eV is a very small quantity of energy: in fact, it would require 1 million electron volts to raise a 1-milligram weight 0.000001 centimeter. Higher-energy photons, such as cosmic rays, have frequencies of 10^{21} hertz (Hz, or cycles per second) or more, and energies of 10^7 eV or more; lower-energy photons, such as those associated with electric and magnetic fields, have frequencies of $10–10^3$ Hz and energies only a tiny fraction of an eV. Photons in the intermediate energy range (10^{-3}–3 eV), such as those associated with infrared and visible light, have frequencies of 10^{12}–10^{15} Hz. Only intermediate-range electromagnetic radiation can be detected by the human senses. High-energy photons are extremely penetrating and can have effects far from their source; the effects of lower-energy photons are concentrated near the source. Figure 9.1 shows the types and energies of the various parts of the

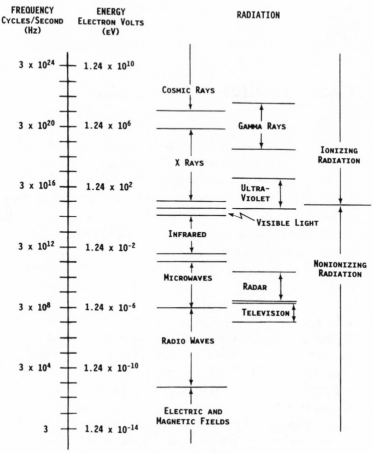

Figure 9.1   The electromagnetic spectrum

electromagnetic spectrum. The energy ranges for the various types of radiation have not been precisely defined in every case; overlaps are common.

As it moves through space, electromagnetic radiation interacts with the atoms composing matter. Photons in the higher-energy ranges, such as X and gamma rays, can ionize these atoms by interacting with the orbital electrons and stripping them away. Under normal circumstances, an atom is electrically neutral, having the same number of negatively charged electrons in orbit as it has positive charges (protons) in its nucleus. Once an electron is removed, it exhibits a unit negative charge, and the residual atom shows a net unit positive charge. These two products are known as an ion pair (Figure 9.2). This transfer of energy to atoms can result in chemical and biological changes that are harmful to health.

To remove an electron from an atom, and thus create an ion pair, requires theoretically at least 10 eV. Since much of the energy expended by photons in interacting with matter does not result in ionization, the average energy required to produce an ion pair is much larger, about 34 eV. Only the photons associated with cosmic, X, and gamma rays and with the higher-frequency ultraviolet radiation possess this amount of energy. These are the only portions of the electromagnetic spectrum that are *ionizing*. Photons associated with

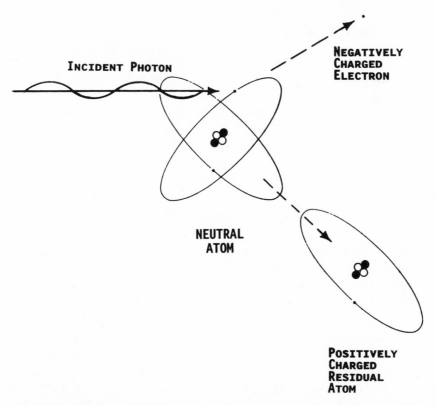

Figure 9.2   Interaction of X or gamma photon with a neutral atom to produce an ion pair

the lower-energy portions of the spectrum, ranging from lower-energy ultraviolet radiation down through infrared, radar, radio, and the electric and magnetic fields associated with many household appliances and electric power lines, are *nonionizing*. However, these types of radiation also have associated health effects.

Nonionizing Radiation

Although the biological effects of ionizing radiation have been recognized and reasonably understood for some time, questions remain concerning the effects of certain types of nonionizing radiation, in particular the photons associated with lower-energy electric and magnetic fields. Techniques for assessing radiation from many such sources are still evolving.

Ultraviolet Radiation

The major natural source of ultraviolet (UV) radiation is the sun. Artificial sources include electric arcs used in lights, welding arcs, plasma jets, germicidal lamps, and special tanning lamps. The amount of UV radiation reaching the earth from the sun depends on factors such as the season, time of day, latitude, amount of cloud cover, condition of the protective ozone layer, and elevation above sea level. At higher elevations there is more UV radiation because there is less atmosphere between the earth and the sun. The amount of UV radiation received can also be increased by radiation reflected from water, snow, or sand. Such exposure can result in snow or sun "blindness."

UV radiation is unable to penetrate most materials and so is readily shielded. Ordinary window glass will remove most of the higher frequencies, and a light layer of clothing will eliminate essentially all frequencies. Since the biological effects of UV radiation do not appear until some time after exposure has occurred, people can receive an excessive amount before becoming aware of the extent of the damage. If the exposure is sufficiently high, there may be marked systemic effects, including fever, nausea, and malaise. Aging of the skin also appears to be closely related with cumulative exposure to UV radiation. In the areas of highest exposure, premalignant or malignant changes may develop. For this reason the International Radiation Protection Association has issued recommendations for the control of exposures from sun lamps and from ultraviolet lamps such as those used in tanning booths (1991).

Some people are particularly sensitive to UV radiation because their skin has relatively little pigmentation. Others may be sensitive as a result of specific diseases, such as xeroderma pigmentosa, lupus erythematosus, pellagra, and porphyria, that lead to photosensitivity. Farm workers may develop a sensitivity to UV radiation as a result of contact with molds growing in certain plants. Fungi growing in celery, for example, produce psoralen, a chemical that photosynthesizes the skin. A number of medications and plant extracts can also produce photosensitivity. People can protect themselves against UV radiation by wearing dark glasses and clothing and by applying creams containing chemicals that absorb radiation in this energy range.

Visible Light (including Lasers)

The health effects of visible light may be direct or indirect. An example of the former is a retinal burn from looking at the sun with inadequate filtration during an eclipse; an example of the latter is injury from an accident caused by inadequate or excessive lighting. Inadequate lighting can result in a fall; excessive lighting, such as the glare of the headlights of an oncoming car, can cause a crash.

Other health problems are associated with the use of devices in which beams of light can be focused both temporally and spatially. These devices, called lasers (for *l*ight *a*mplification by *s*timulated *e*mission of *r*adiation), have found a wide range of industrial, consumer, scientific, and medical applications. These include alignment of tunnels, distance measurement, welding, cutting, drilling, heat treatment, entertainment (laser light shows), and surgery. Lasers are also used in video disc players, supermarket scanners, and facsimile and printing equipment. In most such applications, laser units are totally or partially enclosed to prevent exposure to direct or scattered radiation.

Because laser devices have extremely small divergence and their beams are highly collimated, they are highly directional and can be focused on a spot whose diameter is equal to about one wavelength of the emitted light. As a result, extraordinarily high temperatures can be generated in the small area where the radiation is absorbed. Even minute quantities of laser light can burn a small hole in the retina and impair vision permanently. Standards for protective eyewear for industrial laser users have been developed by the American National Standards Institute (Tanner, 1990). The lenses of protective eyewear can be either reflective or absorptive. Many reflective filters are made of glass with a thin surface coating. Glass filters can generally withstand a higher heat and energy load than most plastics. Their disadvantage is that a scratch in the lens may allow radiation to penetrate to the eye. Absorptive filters are now being designed to diffuse the incoming laser energy harmlessly across the lens.

Infrared Radiation

All objects emit infrared radiation to other objects that have a lower surface temperature. The higher the temperature, the higher the frequency and energy of the radiation. With extremely high temperatures, the energies of the emissions can move from the infrared into the visible-light portion and even into the lower ranges of the UV portion of the spectrum. This change has been incorporated in the language of the iron and steel industry: "white hot" is hotter than "red hot."

One example of infrared radiation is the heat from the sun. Another is the heat produced by a stove or by the radiant heating units used in many dwellings. Fortunately, the sensation of heat is quickly detected and thus provides adequate warning of extreme conditions. Infrared radiation does not penetrate deeply into skin tissues, but if not controlled it can cause burns on the skin, cataracts in the lens of the eye (which has poor heat-dissipating mechanisms), or retinal damage. Infrared sources can so increase the thermal load on people that their sweating mechanisms cannot provide adequate cooling. High body temperature may result in heat stroke or heat exhaustion; excessive loss of salt through perspiration may cause heat cramps.

Since infrared radiation is readily reflected by polished surfaces, people can protect themselves against localized sources by special clothing and shielding. In buildings, air-conditioning and ventilation systems can dissipate excess heat to the outdoor environment.

Microwaves

Microwave radiation sources include radar, radio and television transmitters, satellite telecommunication systems, and, of course, microwave ovens. In industry, microwaves are used to dry and cure ply-wood, paint, inks, and synthetic rubber and to control insects in stored grain. In medicine, microwaves provide deep-heat therapy for the relief of aching joints and sore muscles, and they have been used to reheat blood rapidly after certain types of surgery (G. T. Johnson, 1982).

Microwaves are reflected by metal; they pass through glass, paper, and plastic; and they are readily absorbed by materials containing water. In microwave ovens, microwaves agitate the water molecules, and the resulting molecular friction produces heat. The effects of microwaves in living organisms, however, appear to be more complex than simple heating, although most of the changes can be attributed to this phenomenon. Because the tissues in the human body vary in electrical conductance, capacitance, inductance, and resonance, there are large differences in their absorption of microwave radiation. Furthermore, as the energy passes from a tissue of one conductivity to another, reflections and standing waves may develop that can alter the effects (Ferris, 1966).

Microwaves have frequencies of 10^8–10^{11} Hz. The body is largely transparent to the lower frequencies ($<1.5 \times 10^8$ Hz), and microwaves in this energy range produce no biological effects. As frequency increases above this range, however, the energy of microwaves is increasingly absorbed, reaching a maximum at about 3×10^8 Hz, in the ultra-high-frequency (UHF) television range. At still higher frequencies ($>10^9$ Hz), less of the energy is absorbed, and above 10^{10} Hz the skin acts as a reflector. The frequency range 10^8–10^9 Hz is potentially the most hazardous because within it there is little or no heating of the skin and the thermal receptors are not stimulated. In contrast, higher-energy microwaves ($>10^9$ Hz) interact with the skin, producing a sensation of warmth that provides prompt warning of their presence. Above 10^{10} Hz, microwaves are either reflected by the skin, or absorbed in only the superficial layers, and the effects are minimal (Ferris, 1966).

The testes and eyes appear to be the most vulnerable to the heating effects of microwave radiation. A man exposed directly to a microwave beam and close to its source may experience temporary sterility. The eye, with its poor blood supply, particularly around the lens, is susceptible to cataract formation, especially for microwaves in the energy range 2.5–3×10^9 Hz, which can penetrate to that depth (Ferris, 1966). Sufficient exposure can also produce thermal burns in the skin and eyes. Exposures to high-power densities in the wave guide of a microwave transmitter can be lethal.

Electric and Magnetic Fields

The flow of electricity through wires produces electric and magnetic fields. High-voltage electric power transmission lines are probably the most publicized sources of such fields; there are more than 300,000 miles of these lines in the United States today. But many consumer products are also sources of electric and magnetic fields. These include electric blankets, electric toasters, microwave ovens, hair dryers, television sets, and desktop computers (Moore, 1990).

The primary concern today, the health effects of magnetic fields, developed first in the late 1960s, when controversy arose over the potential health effects associated with high-voltage transmission lines. Since then the Electric Power Research Institute (EPRI) has conducted extensive studies on the subject (Shepard, 1987; EPRI, 1989; Moore, 1990). In 1988 the Congressional Office of Technology Assessment (OTA) also commissioned a detailed review of relevant information (Nair, Morgan, and Florig, 1989). The EPRI review concluded that although the possibility that magnetic fields play a role in carcinogenesis cannot be ruled out, no carcinogenic mechanism has yet been identified. Nor has there been an accurate assessment of human risk. Although several epidemiologic studies suggest a weak association between exposure to low-frequency magnetic fields and increased risk of various kinds of cancer, the magnitude of the increased risk was usually small, and the findings of the studies were inconsistent. According to the OTA report, if exposures to magnetic fields do affect human health, the major problem area will be the use of electricity in households. Toasters and electric blankets, for example, produce electric and magnetic fields comparable to those near the right-of-way of many high-voltage transmission lines (Nair, Morgan, and Florig, 1989).

The cancer-promoting mechanisms of magnetic fields have been studied indirectly in cells and tissues; however, the carcinogenic effects of such fields on animals have not been directly addressed. Some studies suggest that electric and magnetic fields may affect the immune and endocrine systems or growth-regulatory signals, possibly as a result of changes in the flow of calcium through cell membranes. A number of cell types have shown increased cell growth, cell division, and transcription. Many bioeffects have been reported to occur only with certain specific combinations of frequency, amplitude, and orientation of the electromagnetic radiation signal with respect to the geomagnetic field. If this implied complex dose-response relationship does exist, evaluating the risk of electric and magnetic field exposures on human health will be very difficult (EPRI, 1989). Careful studies are needed to determine whether the effects of electric and magnetic fields are related to the average exposure over a period of time, to infrequent exposures to very high fields, to changes in the fields, or to some combination of these and other factors (Abelson, 1989).

Standards for Control

Guidelines on limits for occupational exposures to ultraviolet, laser, infrared, and microwave radiation and for static magnetic fields have been published by the American Conference of Governmental Industrial Hygienists (ACGIH, 1990). Limits for exposures from the use of microwave ovens have been established by the U.S. Department of Health and Human Services (1970). Limits for exposures of workers and the general public to a wide range of nonionizing electromagnetic radiation have been published by the International Radiation Protection Association (IRPA, 1985a, 1985b, 1988; Duchene and Lakey, 1990). Many of the limits are complex, because of the different effects of various electromagnetic radiation as a function of energy. In many cases the recommendations are based largely on value judgments because the only data available were from experiments with animals. For this reason, a variety of cautionary statements accompany the standards, particularly those published by the ACGIH. These include general warnings that none of the standards should be regarded "as representing a fine line between safe and dangerous levels" and that "needless exposure to all radiofrequency radiation exposures should be avoided given the current state of knowledge on human effects, particularly nonthermal effects." The standards also caution that the limits for UV radiation "do not apply to individuals concomitantly exposed to photosensitizing agents," and that the standards for magnetic radiation must be reduced for workers who have implanted cardiac pacemakers (because of the possibility of interference with their operation) (ACGIH, 1990). Further research on the biological effects of these environmental factors is obviously needed.

In its standards for ultraviolet radiation, the IRPA sought to prevent skin erythema (reddening) as well as potential delayed effects such as skin cancer and cataracts. In its considerations of laser radiation, the association recognized that this technology is finding increasing use in consumer and office devices and that, within the optical spectrum, there are enormous variations in biological effects, particularly in the different structures of the eye potentially at risk. In its assessment of electromagnetic fields, the IRPA noted the need to limit peak values for pulsed as well as for continuous fields. It also noted that the presence of humans distorts the field and changes the nature of the exposures and that exposures are not limited to the workplace. The possibility that the general public may be exposed in many settings imposes other restrictions. For example, because they are smaller, children have a higher absorption rate for higher-frequency electromagnetic fields, and the distribution of energy absorption in various body parts is different. For these reasons, exposure limits for the general public have been set much lower than for occupationally exposed workers. The same approach has been used in setting limits for exposures to ionizing radiation (Chapter 10).

Although the risks from exposures to electric and magnetic fields are thought to be small, there is sufficient information to mandate a cautious approach before permitting widespread and unnecessary exposures to such sources. In fact, in anticipation of the possible confirmation of biological effects the EPRI has initiated a program to develop methods for reducing exposures from electric and magnetic fields associated with both the transmission and use of electricity (Hidy, 1990).

Ionizing Radiation

Ionizing radiation is produced by photons with high enough energy to ionize atoms. It includes X rays, discovered by Wilhelm Roentgen in 1895; and alpha, beta, and gamma rays, first observed when Antoine Henri Becquerel discovered naturally radioactive materials in 1896. The environment contains a host of naturally occurring radioactive materials, most of which are derived from the decay of uranium. Much lower levels of artificially produced radioactive materials have been discharged into the environment as a result of atmospheric weapons tests and the operation of nuclear facilities.

Interaction with Matter

Through its ability to penetrate cells and to deposit energy among atoms in a random manner, ionizing radiation creates changes that can lead to biological damage. These changes include the production of toxic agents such as free radicals and hydrogen peroxide, which are formed by the ionization of water molecules in cells. Both the direct effects (deposition of energy and creation of ion pairs) and the indirect effects (subsequent production of toxic agents) of radiation can interfere with normal life processes. All cells are susceptible to damage by ionizing radiation, and only a very small amount of energy needs to be deposited in a cell or tissue to produce significant biological changes. For example, if all the energy deposited were converted to heat, a dose of radiation to the whole body sufficient to be lethal to human beings would raise the temperature of the body by only 0.001°C. Fortunately, ionizing radiation can be measured accurately at exposure levels several orders of magnitude below those required to produce measurable biological effects in human cells (Little, 1986).

Units of Dose

On the basis of developing knowledge about the deposition of energy and its associated biological effects, units have been evolved to express the doses that result from exposures to ionizing radiation (Table 9.1). The one most commonly used today is the unit of equivalent dose, the sievert (Sv), although an earlier unit, the rem, is still in use in some parts of the world. One Sv is equal to 100 rem. Both units are a measure of the amount, distribution, and resulting biological effects of the ions created by the passage of radiation through tissue. Since both units represent larger doses than are usually encountered in the workplace and the ambient environment, subunits have been developed. The most common of these is the millisievert (mSv). One mSv is equal to 100 millirem (mrem).

Table 9.1 Units of dose for ionizing radiation (historical development)

Unit	Description
Roentgen	The roentgen, now obsolete, was first introduced at the Radiological Congress held in Stockholm in 1928 as the special unit for expressing exposure to ionizing radiation. It was based on the quantity of electrical charge produced in air by X or gamma radiation. One roentgen (r) of exposure will produce about 2 billion ion pairs per cubic centimeter of air.
Rad	The rad was first defined by the International Commission on Radiation Units and Measurements (ICRU) in 1953 as the special unit of absorbed dose. It was developed to reflect the fact that the exposure of soft tissue or similar material to 1 r results in the absorption of about 100 ergs of energy per gram (1 rad). The *r*adiation *a*bsorbed *d*ose served for many years as the standard unit of dose.
Rem	When the biological effects of ionizing radiation were found to depend on the nature of the radiation, as well as on other factors, a unit was needed for expressing the effects of all types of ionizing radiation on a biologically equivalent basis. The *r*oentgen *e*quivalent *m*an, or rem, which was introduced by the ICRU in 1962, is equal to the absorbed dose in rad multiplied by the appropriate Radiation-Weighting Factor. For X or gamma radiation, the Radiation-Weighting Factor is one. Thus, 1 rad of absorbed dose from X or gamma radiation is equal to 1 rem. Similarly, 1 rad of absorbed dose from beta radiation is equal to 1 rem. For alpha radiation, 1 rad equals 20 rem (the Radiation Weighting Factor in this case having a value of 20).
Gray	Following the International System of Units, the General Conference on Weights and Measures (CGPM, from the initials of the French name) replaced the rad in 1975 with the gray, the unit of *absorbed dose*. One gray (Gy) is equal to 100 rad.
Sievert	Following the International System of Units, the CGPM replaced the rem in 1977 with the sievert, the unit of *equivalent dose* (often called simply the *dose*). One sievert (Sv) is equal to 100 rem; one millisievert (mSv) is equal to 100 millirem (mrem).

Classification of Exposures

On the basis of the total dose and the dose rate, the effects of radiation exposures can be classified as either *deterministic* or *stochastic* (ICRP, 1991a). Deterministic effects are those for which the severity of the effect varies with the dose, and for which a threshold may therefore occur. Stochastic effects are those for which the probability that an effect will occur, rather than the severity of the effect, is regarded as a function of the dose, without threshold. Deterministic effects are generally associated with *acute* exposures involving doses in the range of tens of sievert delivered to part or all of the body over a short period. Deterministic effects include cataracts, sterility, tissue damage (for example, erythema), and death (Table 9.2). Most stochastic effects are the result of *chronic* exposures (the type most commonly encountered in the workplace and the ambient environment) involving repeated low doses to all or part of the body over a period of years. Stochastic effects include cancers (such as leukemia and solid tumors) and genetic damage, manifested in blood abnormalities, metabolic diseases, and physical abnormalities in the exposed person's descendants. Only in situations such as a nuclear war or a major accident at a nuclear facility would one expect to observe any of the acute (deterministic) effects of ionizing radiation.

Dose-Response Relationships

Many studies of human populations, other animals, and cell cultures provide a reliable basis for quantitative estimates of the effects of chronic radiation exposures received at low dose rates. Epidemiologic studies have focused on cancers and genetic damage in survivors of the World War II atomic bombings in Japan; lung cancer in uranium miners exposed underground to airborne radon and its decay products; bone cancer in young women who ingested radium and thorium while painting luminous markings on the faces of clocks and watches; breast cancer in women with tuberculosis who had multiple fluoroscopic chest examinations; and leukemia in patients treated with radiation for ankylosing spondylitis of the spine.

On the basis of these and other studies, several models have been suggested for estimating the relationship between the dose from a radiation source and its effects (Figure 9.3). In general, mutations

Table 9.2   Biological effects on humans of acute whole-body
external doses of ionizing radiation

Equivalent dose		
Sievert	Rem	Effects
0–0.25	0–25	No detectable clinical effects; small increase in risk of delayed cancer and genetic effects
0.25–1	25–100	Slight transient reductions in lymphocytes and neutrophils; sickness not common; long-term effects possible, but serious effects on average individual highly improbable
1–2	100–200	Minimal symptoms; nausea and fatigue with possible vomiting; reduction in lymphocytes and neutrophils, with delayed recovery
2–3	200–300	Nausea and vomiting on first day; following latent period of up to 2 weeks, symptoms (loss of appetite and general malaise) appear but are not severe; recovery likely in about 3 months unless complicated by previous poor health
3–6	300–600	Nausea, vomiting, and diarrhea in first few hours, followed by latent period as long as 1 week with no definite symptoms; loss of appetite, general malaise, and fever during second week, followed by hemorrhage, purpura, inflammation of mouth and throat, diarrhea, and emaciation in third week; some deaths in 2–6 weeks; possible eventual death to 50% of those exposed
6–10	600–1,000	Vomiting in 100% of victims within first few hours; diarrhea, hemorrhage, fever, etc., toward end of first week; rapid emaciation; certain death unless heroic medical treatment is available and successful
10–50	1,000–5,000	Vomiting within 5–30 minutes; 100% incidence of death within 2–14 days
> 50	> 5,000	Vomiting immediately; 100% incidence of death within a few hours to 2 days

induced by radiation in cultured human cells follow a linear model (graph A). In contrast, cell death is related exponentially to dose (graph B). Further complicating the situation is that the shape of the curve appears to vary with the nature of the ionizing radiation. After considerable debate, the Committee on the Biological Effects of Ionizing Radiation of the National Research Council (BEIR, 1980) suggested that for X and gamma rays, the data appeared to support a relationship combining the linear and quadratic models (graph C). Although newer data appear to support this conclusion with regard to the induction of leukemia, it now appears that the induction of solid tumors (cancers of the thyroid, breast, and bone) follows a linear model (BEIR, 1990).

One reason for the continuing controversy about the quantitative relationship between doses from ionizing radiation and their associated health effects is that the sample sizes required for definitive proof are simply unavailable: the necessary sample sizes become prohibitively large when doses are small. For example, to establish firmly the existence of a linear relationship between a radiation dose of 1 Sv and the risk of lung cancer would require 1,000 subjects who had received that dose; to establish such a relationship at a dose of 0.1 Sv would require 100,000 people who had received that dose; and to do so at 0.01 Sv would require a sample of 10 million subjects (Shore, 1991).

The choice of a model can radically affect estimates of the effects of ionizing radiation. If the dose-response curve is assumed to be linear (Figure 9.3, graph A) for solid tumors, as the latest analyses

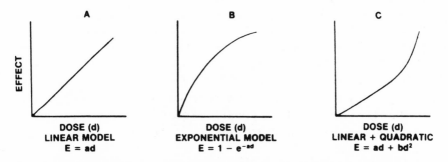

Figure 9.3   Dose-response models for quantifying the effects of ionizing radiation

indicate, then incremental increases in the effects produced by any dose will be similar in the high- and low-dose ranges. In fact, if the induction of solid tumors follows a linear relationship, the likelihood of a person's becoming ill with cancer after being exposed to a given dose of radiation will be three to four times greater than if the dose-response relationship follows a linear quadratic relationship. The assumption of a linear relationship for the induction of solid tumors and leukemia also implies that however low the dose is, there may be some health effect, however small.

Types of Exposures

Both external and internal exposures from ionizing radiation are potential threats to human health in the workplace and in the general environment.

External Exposures

Regardless of the assumptions regarding the dose-response model, for sources of ionizing radiation external to the body the resulting injury will depend on (1) the total dose, (2) the dose rate, and (3) the percentage and region of the body exposed. In general, the potential for harmful effects increases along with increases in these three factors. The major concern in the protection of both radiation workers and the general public is the probability of stochastic effects, primarily latent cancers.

Internal Exposures

Internal exposures result from the presence or deposition of radioactive materials in the body through ingestion or inhalation. The potential for harm depends on the types and quantities of material taken in and how long they remain in the body. For example, materials that emit alpha particles represent a greater hazard than those that emit beta particles. In general, the greater the quantity of radioactive material consumed and the longer it remains in the body, the greater the hazard.

The International Commission on Radiological Protection and the National Council on Radiation Protection and Measurements have developed annual limits on intake for a large number of radioactive materials (ICRP 1991b). For radionuclides that distribute rather uniformly throughout the body, the permissible intake is calculated on the basis of the equivalent dose limit for the whole body. For radionuclides that concentrate predominantly in a single organ, the annual limit on intake is based on the concept of effective dose (Chapter 10). To protect people from airborne radionuclides, the annual limits on intake have been converted to equivalent derived air concentrations. Similar calculations have been made for drinking water. Both have been incorporated in the regulations of the U.S. Nuclear Regulatory Commission (NRC) and the Occupational Safety and Health Administration. Techniques for monitoring various avenues of intake to assure compliance with these regulations include analyses of food, water, and air, as well as bioassay and whole-body counting procedures. Techniques also exist for monitoring the movement of radioactive materials in the environment and for estimating doses to members of the public (Chapter 11).

Natural Background Radiation

Human beings have always been exposed to a significant level of radiation from natural sources, in the forms of cosmic radiation from outer space, external radiation from naturally occurring radioactive materials in the earth, and internal radiation from radioactive materials taken into the body in water, food, and air. Because these natural sources constitute the overwhelming majority of radiation exposure to people throughout the world, and because the exposures have persisted for millennia, knowledge of the associated dose rates should be helpful both for understanding the effects of ionizing radiation and for setting acceptable limits for radiation exposures from artificial sources.

Today the annual dose from cosmic radiation at sea level is about 0.3–0.35 mSv. Since the atmosphere serves as a shield against cosmic radiation, this dose increases with altitude. At an altitude of 1 mile, the annual dose from cosmic radiation is about double that at sea level; at 12,000 feet it is about 1 mSv; at 40,000 feet (where subsonic aircraft routinely operate) it is 15–20 mSv; and at 80,000 feet (where supersonic aircraft operate) it can approach 60–80 mSv. Since passengers on a flight across the United States are airborne only a few hours, the actual increase in dose through exposure to cosmic radiation is only a few hundredths of a mSv. Although dose rates in supersonic aircraft are higher than those in subsonic aircraft, the total dose for a given trip is about the same, since the supersonic aircraft makes the flight in a much shorter time.

Dose rates from terrestrial sources vary according to the quantities of naturally occurring radioactive materials in the earth; they range from as low as a few tenths of a mSv to as high as several mSv per year. Figure 9.4 shows three major regions of variation. The regions with the highest dose rates are those associated with uranium deposits in the Colorado Plateau, granitic deposits in New England, and phosphate deposits in Florida; those with the lowest rates are the sandy soils of the Atlantic and Gulf coastal plain.

Clearly, the doses that people receive from terrestrial sources vary according to where they live. They also vary according to the amount of naturally occurring radioactive material that people ingest. The principal naturally occurring radionuclides involved are potassium and radium.

Potassium

A common source of potassium is the banana, and one of its isotopes, K-40, is radioactive. Since potassium preferentially deposits in muscular tissue, this radionuclide is widely distributed throughout the body. It contributes an annual dose of about 0.15 mSv to women and about 0.19 mSv to men. Because some of the radiation emitted by potassium is highly penetrating, the potassium in our bodies also exposes people nearby, the associated dose rates being estimated at 0.01–0.02 mSv per year. Potassium in the body is under homeostatic control, and the maintenance of a potassium balance is essential to health. Commercial products such as Gatorade, which contains relatively large quantities of potassium, are specifically designed to restore the potassium balance in athletes who have exercised and perspired heavily.

Radium

Radium is not essential to the body, and the amounts ingested can be controlled. For the average adult, dose rates from this source to por-

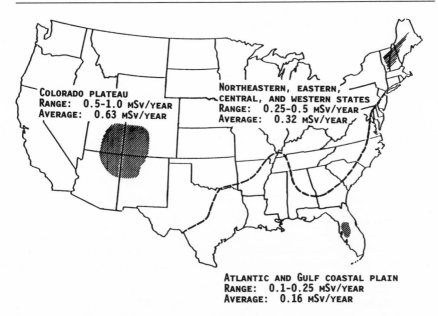

Figure 9.4   Terrestrial dose rates from natural background radiation in the contiguous 48 states

tions of the bone are about 0.17 mSv per year (NCRP, 1987a). For selected population groups, the dose rates can be much higher. Well water in some areas (such as Illinois), for example, contains relatively high concentrations of radium.

One of the most significant sources of radium is the Brazil nut. These nuts, which grow only in the Amazon basin, contain high concentrations of radium because Brazil nut trees need barium but take up radium as a substitute. Concentrations of radium in Brazil nuts average 1–2 picocuries per gram. Some samples of Brazil nuts have been found to contain up to 4 picocuries per gram (Penna-Franca et al., 1968). However, no one is known to have suffered harmful radiation effects from eating Brazil nuts.

Overall, the average nonsmoker in the United States today receives an estimated 3 mSv per year of whole-body equivalent dose from natural radiation sources. As Table 9.3 shows, this accounts for more than 80 percent of the total exposure. Figure 9.5 shows the relative contributions of the principal sources of ionizing radiation in the

Table 9.3   Average annual effective dose of ionizing radiation to nonsmokers,
United States

Source	Dose	
	mSv	mrem
Natural sources		
Radon	2.0	200
Cosmic, terrestrial, internal	1.0	100
Medical		
X-ray diagnosis	0.39	39
Nuclear medicine	0.14	14
Consumer products	~0.1	~10
Occupational	~0.01	~1
Miscellaneous environmental sources	< 0.001	< 0.1
Nuclear fuel cycle	< 0.001	< 0.1
Total	3.6	360

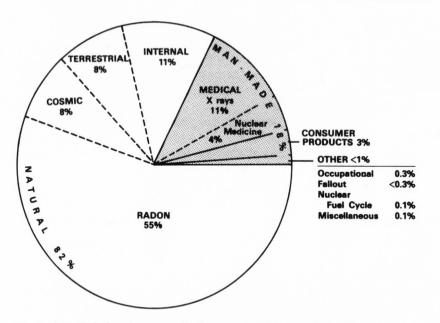

Figure 9.5   Relative dose contributions to the U.S. population from the
principal sources of ionizing radiation

United States. About 55 percent of the total dose comes from the inhalation of radon and its airborne decay products inside buildings (Chapter 2) (NCRP, 1987a, 1987b).

Artificial Sources

Today radiation machines and radioactive materials produced in particle accelerators and nuclear reactors are the principal artificial sources of ionizing radiation.

Radiation Machines

X-ray machines are in widespread use in industry, medicine, commerce, and research. All are potential sources of exposures.

MEDICAL AND DENTAL USES

Estimates are that more than 1 billion diagnostic medical X-ray examinations, more than 300 million dental X-ray examinations, and about 4 million radiation therapy procedures or courses of treatment are performed worldwide each year (Mettler et al., 1987). In the United States about 140,000 X-ray units are used by physicians, chiropractors, and veterinarians for medical diagnosis; more than 200,000 additional units are used by dentists. Figure 9.6 shows the increase in the number of medical and dental X-ray units over the past 40 years. In the period 1964–1980 the number of medical and dental X-ray examinations increased by 72 percent, sales of X-ray film by 152 percent.

Some 800,000–1,000,000 medical and dental personnel are occupationally exposed in the operation of these units. Procedures for protecting them include limiting the time of exposure, maintaining an adequate distance between the X-ray beam and the operator, and providing adequate shielding. Generally, a combination of these three safety principles can restrict doses to acceptable levels. The average occupational exposure of medical and dental X-ray personnel is well below 5 mSv per year, and essentially all of them receive an annual dose less than 10 mSv. Estimates are that the average annual effective dose to workers in the developed countries is 0.1–3 mSv, with the annual collective dose being about 1 person-Sv per million people (Mettler et al., 1990). The collective dose, a unit designed to represent

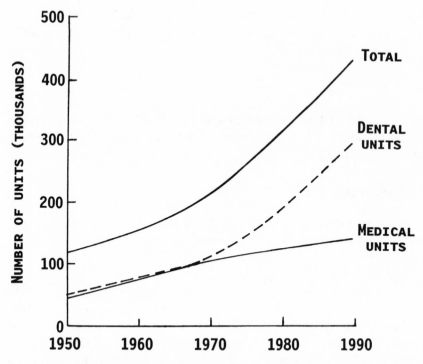

Figure 9.6   Increase in the number of medical and dental X-ray units in the
United States, 1950–1990

the integrated population dose, is equal to the product of the number
of people exposed (expressed in units of persons) times their average
individual dose (expressed in units of sievert) (see Chapter 10).

An estimated 65 percent of Americans visit their doctor or dentist
annually and undergo some type of X-ray procedure. Vigorous programs launched in the early 1960s to control patient exposures (similar
to those used for X-ray unit operators) have kept the increase in doses
far below the increase in the use of X rays. Under these programs, the
federal government promulgated manufacturing standards for medical
and dental X-ray machines; and federal, state, and local regulatory
agencies developed ongoing inspection programs to assure that X-ray
units are operated at the proper voltage, that X-ray beams are properly filtered and collimated, and that physicians and dentists use faster
films and proper processing techniques. Filtration of the beam re-

moves the softer X rays that would otherwise be absorbed by the patient. Proper filtration can reduce the dose to the reproductive organs by 200–500 percent. Proper collimation can reduce the dose to the reproductive organs by a factor of 200 to 500. Progress in reducing the doses from medical and dental X-ray machines was particularly significant during the first two decades of the federal and state control programs. In the years 1964–1983 the average X-ray beam dose at the skin entrance for chest X rays was reduced 25 percent, from 0.28 to 0.21 mSv; and for dental bitewings the skin entrance dose was reduced 76 percent, from 11.5 to 3 mSv. In the same period the beam size of most units used for taking chest X rays was reduced to the size of the film being used, and the diameter of the beams in over 90 percent of dental X-ray units was reduced to 2.75 inches or less, the size considered acceptable for making a dental X-ray film (Johnson and Goetz, 1985).

Reflecting the success of these efforts, the estimated mean dose to the bone marrow of the average adult American increased by only 13 percent from 1970 to 1980, a period in which the number of medical and dental X-ray machines and the sales of X-ray films were increasing dramatically (NCRP, 1989). Overall, medical and dental X-ray examinations are estimated to contribute 0.39 mSv to the annual effective dose to the U.S. population (NCRP, 1987b).

Worldwide, the collective dose from X-ray diagnosis is estimated to be 2–5 million person-Sv per year. Medical X rays account for 90–95 percent of this dose, dental radiography and nuclear medicine (the use of artificially produced radioactive materials in medical diagnosis and therapy) for the remainder. In the developed countries the collective dose from medical X-ray exposures is estimated to be about 0.001 person-Sv per examination. On this basis, the worldwide annual effective dose per person from X-ray diagnosis is estimated to range between 20 and 50 percent of the dose from natural background radiation (Mettler et al., 1990).

INDUSTRIAL USES

Industrial X-ray devices consist primarily of radiographic and fluoroscopic units used to detect defects in castings, fabricated structures, and welds; and fluoroscopic units used to detect foreign material in items such as food products. Today there are about 10,000 industrial radiographic installations in use in the United States; some 40,000–50,000 people are occupationally exposed in their operation. The primary concern here is the control of exposures to the X-ray machine operators. The same techniques of filtration, coning, shielding, and limiting the time of exposure apply here as in the use of medical X rays.

COMMERCIAL USES OF X RAYS

As of 1950, one of the largest commercial uses of X-ray machines was in fitting shoes; there were about 10,000 such units in operation in the United States. Because health authorities considered the accompanying exposures to be entirely unnecessary, this application was later banned. No units remain in operation today.

Since the 1970s X-ray machines have been used increasingly for the inspection of luggage at airports, as a security measure against aircraft highjackings and bombings; more than 1,000 such units are in operation in U.S. airports today. Although travelers often pass close to these units when entering the boarding area, the advanced design of these systems keeps the accompanying doses extremely low, in the range of a few thousandths of a mSv.

RESEARCH USES

High-voltage X-ray machines and particle accelerators are common equipment in the laboratories of universities and research organizations. More than 1,200 cyclotrons, synchrotrons, van de Graaff generators, and betatrons are in operation in the United States, along with about 3,000 electron microscopes and about 10,000 diffraction units. Modern electron microscopes are shielded to protect the operators, but diffraction units still account for a significant number of radiation injuries (primarily burns on the hands).

Artificially Produced Radioactive Materials

The NRC and state agencies have issued approximately 24,000 licenses for medical, academic, and industrial uses of radioactive materials artificially produced in nuclear reactors. About one-third of these licenses are for the use of radioactive pharmaceuticals in nuclear medicine. Approximately 7 million such procedures are performed annually in the United States for medical diagnosis and therapy, in addition to the millions of diagnostic and therapeutic procedures conducted using X-ray machines. Artificially produced radioactive materials are also used in universities and other institutions for teaching and research. These materials are used by industry in both portable and fixed devices, such as thickness, level, and moisture-density gauges, static eliminators, and gas chromatographs. Artificially produced radioactive materials are also used in the manufacture of smoke detectors, and sealed gamma and neutron sources are used to log wells during exploration for oil and gas (NRC, 1991).

The use of artificially produced radioactive materials in the United States is increasing at the rate of 10–15 percent per year. Seventy to 80 percent of all research at the National Institutes of Health involves such materials. Of the 15 Nobel prizes granted in physiology and medicine from 1975 to 1989, 10 were based on research using radioactive materials.

The population undergoing diagnostic nuclear medicine examinations using artificially produced radioactive materials is, in general, much older than the average patient having diagnostic X rays. At the present time, 75 percent of all nuclear medicine procedures are performed on people aged 45 or older; more than 30 percent are performed on patients 65 or older. The annual per capita effective dose from these procedures in the United States in 1982 was estimated to be 0.14 mSv (NCRP, 1987b). In addition to doses to patients, exposures can occur during the preparation, handling, use, and transport of these materials, and through the release of used materials to the environment. For example, more than 50 percent of patients to whom these materials have been administered dispose of their bodily wastes through direct discharge into sewers.

Nuclear Operations

As of 1990, 113 electricity-generating stations powered by nuclear reactors were operating in the United States (Figure 9.7). In addition, about 75 reactors were being used for training and research; about 70 were operating at various facilities of the U.S. Department of Energy; and almost 200 were in operation or being built for military use as propulsion units in submarines, cruisers, and aircraft carriers.

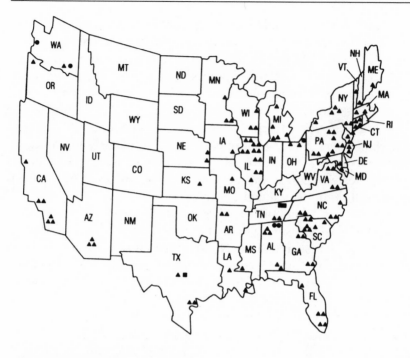

▲ Currently licensed to operate (113)

■ Under construction (3)

● Deferred construction (5)

Figure 9.7   Nuclear power plants in the United States, 1990. There are no commercial reactors in Alaska or Hawaii.

As of 1990 about 425 nuclear power plants, with a total generating capacity of about 300,000 megawatts, were operating worldwide, producing 17 percent of the world's electricity. Eleven nations produce at least one-third of their electricity with nuclear power, and 4 others use it as a major source (France: 75 percent; Belgium: 70 percent; Canada and Sweden: 50 percent). Although nuclear power accounts for only about 20 percent of the electricity generated in the United States, the total amount so generated is larger than in any other country. The worldwide installed capacity for nuclear electricity generation is expected to reach 500,000 megawatts by the year 2000 (Mettler et al., 1990).

Sources of radiation exposure from nuclear power operations include the mining, milling, and fabrication of new fuel; the removal and storage or processing of spent fuel; and the reactor itself.

Mining, Milling, and Fabrication

Several thousand people are employed in uranium mining and milling operations in the United States, mainly in the Colorado Plateau region. There are about 25 uranium mills licensed to operate; another 25 that have been shut down. In addition, there are 21 fuel fabrication plants. At least half of the uranium is now extracted through strip mining, rather than underground mining, resulting in much lower associated radiation exposures to workers. Many of the underground miners, employed during the 1940s and exposed to excessive concentrations of airborne radon and its decay products, have subsequently shown a significant increase in the incidence of lung cancer. During these earlier operations, downstream populations received exposures through ingestion of drinking water contaminated by radium-bearing liquid wastes released from uranium mills. Downwind populations were also exposed to low-level concentrations of radon and its decay products. When the tailings were used as construction materials for the foundations of houses and other buildings, other people in the Colorado Plateau region were exposed to significant concentrations of radon as well as external radiation. Remedial action programs led to the removal of these materials from the buildings.

Both mining and milling operations continue to produce a vast amount of uranium tailings; about 86,000 tons are produced each year in obtaining fuel for the operation of each 1,000-megawatt nuclear power plant (BRWM, 1990). Today there are more than 100 million tons of uranium mill tailings in storage in the United States; about 80 percent of these are located in New Mexico and Wyoming. Tailings stored on the ground surface are being stabilized to control exposures to nearby population groups.

Treatment of Spent Fuel

Each 1,000-megawatt nuclear plant produces about 30 tons of spent fuel each year. In the United States spent fuel from commercial nuclear plants is being held for ultimate disposal in a high-level waste repository. Other countries, such as France, Germany, and Japan, reprocess spent fuel so that the unused uranium and the plutonium, produced in the fuel by the bombardment of uranium with neutrons, can be recycled in nuclear power plants. Reprocessing operations discharge low-level radioactive wastes into the atmosphere and the aquatic environment and produce high-level liquid wastes that must subsequently be solidified for disposal. Although spent fuel from commercial U.S. nuclear power plants is not currently being reprocessed, millions of gallons of high-level liquid wastes from reprocessing of spent fuel from military reactors are now being stored and await solidification prior to emplacement in an underground repository. Through congressional and presidential action, Yucca Mountain, in Nevada, has been selected as the potential location for the first such repository. If the proposed site is found to be acceptable, the first emplacement of high-level wastes is expected to occur in about 20 years (Chapter 6).

Nuclear Reactors

Workers at nuclear power plants receive exposures through radiation from the reactor and from radioactive materials released from it. Data for 1990 show that the collective occupational dose per nuclear power plant in the United States was about 3–4 person-Sv, depending on the type of plant. These data compare favorably with average values of about 6–12 person-Sv for nuclear plants in the United States in 1980 (Institute of Nuclear Power Operations, 1991). Moreover, no worker at any of the plants in 1990 exceeded the annual dose limit of 50 mSv; in fact the average occupational dose for the year was well below 10 mSv. These results reflect the regulatory efforts of the NRC and the activities of the Institute of Nuclear Power Operations, an organization supported by the nuclear industry.

Although the spent fuel contains the bulk of the radioactive material produced in the operation of a nuclear reactor, some radioactive materials leak from the fuel into the cooling system and result in low-level airborne and liquid waste releases. Low-level solid radioactive waste is also produced as a result of various plant operations, as well as in the medical, industrial, and research applications of artificially produced radioactive materials. In 1990 each nuclear power plant in the United States produced an average of 100–300 cubic meters of low-level solid waste, the amount depending on the type of plant. These volumes represent a fourfold to sixfold decrease from the amounts produced in 1980 (Institute of Nuclear Power Operations, 1991). Through the Low Level Radioactive Waste Policy Act, a program is under way for the states, either individually or through compacts, to develop facilities for the disposal of these wastes (Chapter 6).

Environmental releases from nuclear power plants operating in the United States are limited by NRC regulations. For example, Title 10, Part 50, of the Code of Federal Regulations limits the dose rate to the maximally exposed person offsite to about 0.1 mSv per year. In 1987 the total collective dose to the 150 million people living within 50 miles of nuclear power plants in the United States was less than 0.8 person-Sv (NRC, 1990). The average 50-year dose commitment to each person in this group for releases occurring in 1987 ranged from 2×10^{-8} to 9×10^{-5} mSv. The maximum dose during that year for any member of the U.S. population was estimated to be less than 0.01 mSv.

The collective occupational dose per gigawatt-year of electrical energy production associated with all operations performed in the nuclear fuel cycle is estimated to be 12 person-Sv. Offsite populations receive an estimated additional 12 person-Sv from environmental releases associated with uranium mill tailings, nuclear power plant operations, and radioactive waste disposal. The overall annual per-person effective dose worldwide from the nuclear generation of electricity is estimated to be 0.00015 mSv. This exposure is equivalent to 0.01 percent of the annual dose from natural background sources (Mettler et al., 1990).

Radiation Exposures from Consumer Products

A number of natural and artificially produced radioactive materials are used in consumer products and can lead to exposures to members of the public. Such products include luminous clocks and watches, smoke detectors, a variety of glazed and tinted products, and tobacco products.

Luminous Clocks and Watches

During World War II, radium was used to produce luminous paints for the faces of timepieces, compasses, gauges, dials, and other instruments used by the armed forces. After the war many of these products were sold to the public as government surplus items, and some probably remain in use today. With the recognition that such devices could be a significant source of exposure, radium was largely replaced by less-hazardous, artificially produced radioactive materials such as tritium (radioactive hydrogen) and promethium. The last wrist watches incorporating radium were produced in the United States in 1968, the last clocks about 1978.

Estimates of the external whole-body dose rates to people who use radium timepieces range from 0.005 to 0.03 mSv per year. However, localized doses to wearers of radium wristwatches and pocket watches can range up to 3 mSv per year. One study of radium alarm clocks (in which the clock was assumed to have been placed near the user's bed) showed that the resulting annual whole-body doses could range as high as 0.05–0.1 mSv. By contrast, dose rates from timepieces containing tritium and promethium are estimated to be only a few thousandths of a mSv per year (NCRP, 1987c). In fact much of the radiation they emit is absorbed by the watch casing or glass face.

Smoke Detectors

The most widely used smoke detectors in the United States—about 100 million—contain americium, an artificially produced radioactive material. The dose rate from such detectors, which have saved thousands of lives by alerting building occupants to fires, is well below 0.01 mSv per year, an inconsequential amount (NCRP, 1987c).

Glazed and Tinted Products

Eyeglasses tinted with uranium or thorium can produce dose rates of 40 mSv per year to the cornea. False teeth glazed with uranium result in annual dose rates of about 7 mSv to the basal mucosa of the gums of some 45 million denture wearers. "Fiesta-ware" china, which is glazed with uranium, can produce dose rates of 0.1–0.2 mSv per *hour* to diners (Moeller, Hickey, and Schmidt, 1988).

Tobacco Products

Two naturally occurring radioactive materials, lead-210 and polonium-210, are commonly present in tobacco. Both of these longer-lived decay products of radon are deposited and retained on the large, sticky leaves of tobacco plants. When the tobacco is made into cigarettes and the smoker lights up, the radon decay products are volatilized and enter the lungs. The resulting dose to small segments of the bronchial epithelium of the lungs of the approximately 50 million smokers in the United States is estimated to be about 160 mSv per year (NCRP, 1987c). Cigarettes probably represent the single greatest source of radiation exposure to smokers in the United States today. The dose to the whole body equal to this dose to the lungs for a two-pack-per-day smoker is estimated to be about 13 mSv—more than ten times the long-term dose-rate limit for members of the public (Chapter 10).

Control

To be effective, control measures must be practical. Although natural background is the greatest source of radiation exposure, some natural sources are not amenable to control. One example is the dose received from radioactive potassium in the body. Potassium is essential to health, and there is no practical way to avoid the accompanying dose. Much the same can be said for cosmic radiation; it would be impractical for people living in cities such as Denver to move to lower altitudes simply to avoid the dose from this source.

Although airborne radon and its decay products in dwellings represent the largest natural source of radiation exposure, people have been slow to adopt control measures. One major reason is that measures recommended by the EPA require expensive alterations made by an outside contractor. Until homeowners become aware of simpler approaches, such as merely circulating the air inside or using a fan with a positive-ion generator, little progress can be expected (Chapter 2).

The success of control efforts in the medical field is the result of several factors. One is that the U.S. Department of Health and Human Services (HHS) has established standards for the manufacture of diagnostic X-ray machines so they will cause minimal exposure to patients. A second is the vigorous manner in which state health and regulatory agencies, in cooperation with HHS, have pursued programs for the inspection of medical X-ray machines on a regular and continuing basis. Joint federal and state approaches have also been effective in controlling exposures from radioactive materials in medicine and research. All users of significant quantities of such materials must be licensed, and part of the licensing procedure involves a demonstration that applicants have the training, equipment, and facilities to handle such materials safely.

Since it is not yet possible to prove that low doses have no effect, the general approach to the control of radiation sources is to assume that radiation damage has no threshold; that is, however small the dose, it may have some harmful effect. As a result, the current radiation protection philosophy is not only that no one shall receive a dose above the limit, but also that whatever exposures do occur shall be maintained "as low as reasonably achievable." The NRC, for example, requires nuclear power plants to be designed and operated so that waste releases to the environment are only a small fraction of the limits currently recommended by the NCRP and incorporated into federal regulations. Since such restrictions are readily attainable with existing technology, the NRC has made them mandatory.

The control of radioactive materials in industrial, medical, and research applications is largely a function of the form they are in. Control measures for materials sealed in a capsule (for example, for use in radiography) are very similar to those for X-ray machines. Materials in "loose" form, used in laboratory research and nuclear medicine, require careful handling and monitoring. Usually they must be processed only inside a hood (particularly if there is a chance of airborne releases), the handler must wear gloves and a laboratory coat or other protective clothing, and smoking or the consumption of food or drink in the work area is not permitted. In some instances, such as in decontamination operations at nuclear facilities, workers may require extensive protective clothing (boots, head coverings, and respirators).

Control of liquid and airborne radioactive waste may involve containment and isolation, dilution and dispersion, or a combination of the two. For low-volume high-level waste, containment is the only acceptable approach. Dilution and dispersion is generally feasible only for waste with extremely low concentrations of radioactive materials. Intermediate-level waste is often handled by a combination of approaches: the radioactive material content is concentrated and confined and sent to a high-level waste repository, and the decontaminated residual is placed in a low-level waste-disposal facility.

Benefits

Although nonionizing radiation sources have potentially harmful effects, they also improve our standard of living in both small and major ways. Examples include household appliances such as toasters, irons, electric blankets, home computers, and microwave ovens; microwave ovens not only heat and cook foods fast but also use far less electricity than conventional ovens. Radar promotes safety in airline transport. Although the health effects of the electric and magnetic fields associated with high-voltage lines are still not known, transmitting electricity at higher voltages has reduced losses significantly and made electricity and its associated benefits widely available.

Applications of sources of ionizing radiation are also bringing benefits to people throughout the world. Nuclear power, despite its problems, holds promise of generating electricity without accompanying airborne releases of sulfur, nitrogen, and carbon dioxide. The use of X rays in medicine has not only improved the diagnosis of disease but also, in the case of radiation therapy, provided a means for treating cancer. Radiation is also used to sterilize medical supplies, such as surgical gloves and syringes, thus protecting patients and medical personnel against the transmission of infections in hospitals and clinics.

In a similar manner, the use of artificially produced radioactive materials has led to dramatic improvements in medical diagnosis and therapy and related research in physiology and medicine. There are approximately 24,000 nuclear scanners or cameras in use in hospitals worldwide, and nearly 24 million imaging studies are now conducted annually. In the industrialized world, about 25 percent of hospital patients undergo a nuclear medicine procedure during diagnosis or treatment. An estimated 18,000 radiotherapy machines are in use worldwide, with about 5 million patients being treated annually (Blix, 1989).

Controls using radioactive materials for monitoring the operation of machines are widely used in industry. Thickness gauges, in particular, have led to improved quality control of manufactured goods. Nucleonic systems are now used to control entire processes in the steel and coal industries. In the paper industry, such systems control both thickness and moisture content, saving materials and energy (Blix, 1989).

In agriculture, nuclear techniques such as gamma or neutron irradiation have been used to induce mutations in seeds and thus create new varieties of food crops. In 1960 there were 15 radiation-induced mutant varieties available to growers; today there are more than 1,300, bred for higher yield, better quality, and improved resistance to disease and pests. Sixty percent of the durum wheat grown in Italy to produce pasta is a gamma-induced mutant variety. In China about 8 million hectares (almost 10 percent of China's cultivated land) are planted with strains of rice produced through radiation-induced mutations, yielding crops valued at an estimated $1 billion annually (Blix, 1989).

The use of radionuclides in agricultural research has also brought many benefits. For example, an isotope of nitrogen has been used to identify the best way of applying nitrogen fertilizers in rice production, reducing the quantity required by up to 50 percent. In addition to economic savings, there is less runoff of surplus nitrogen compounds into groundwater, rivers, and lakes.

Radiation is also being used to control insects such as the screwworm fly, the Mediterranean fruit fly, and the tse-tse fly. Radiation at the pupa stage produces sterile but otherwise normal adults that are released into the environment and mate but produce no offspring (Chapter 7).

Finally, radiation is being used in 36 countries, including the United States, to preserve food. Worldwide, some 40 different food items, including spices, grains, chicken, meat, fruits, and vegetables, have been approved for preservation by this method (Chapter 5).

References

Abelson, Philip H. 1989. "Effects of Electric and Magnetic Fields." Editorial. *Science* 245, no. 4915 (21 July), 241.
ACGIH. 1990. *1990–1991 Threshold Limit Values for Chemical Substances and Physical Agents and Biological Exposure Indices.* Cincinnati.
BEIR. 1980. *The Effects on Populations of Exposure to Low Levels of Ionizing Radiation.* Report no. III. Washington, D.C.: National Academy Press.
——— 1990. *Health Effects of Exposure to Low Levels of Ionizing Radiation.* Report no. V. Washington, D.C.: National Academy Press.

Blix, H. 1989. "The Peaceful Applications of Nuclear Energy." Paper presented at the annual symposium of the Uranium Institute, London, 6–8 September.

BRWM. 1990. *Rethinking High-Level Radioactive Waste Management*. Washington, D.C.: National Academy Press.

Duchene, A. S., and John Lakey, eds. 1990. *The IRPA Guidelines on Protection against Non-Ionizing Radiation*. New York: Pergamon Press.

EPRI. 1989. *Extremely Low Frequency Electric and Magnetic Fields and Cancer: A Literature Review*. Report EPRI EN-6674. Palo Alto.

Ferris, Benjamin G. 1966. "Environmental Hazards: Electromagnetic Radiation." *New England Journal of Medicine* 275 (17 November), 1100–05.

Hidy, George M. 1990. "EMG Research: A Commitment to Excellence." Editorial. *EPRI Journal* 15, no. 1 (January/February), 1.

ICRP. 1991a. *1990 Recommendations of the International Commission on Radiological Protection*. Publication 60, Annals of the ICRP, vol. 21, no. 1–3. New York: Pergamon Press.

———— 1991b. *Annual Limits on Intake of Radionuclides by Workers Based on the 1990 Recommendations*. Publication 61, Annals of the ICRP, vol. 21, no. 4. New York: Pergamon Press.

IRPA. International Non-Ionizing Radiation Committee. 1985a. "Guidelines on Limits of Exposure to Ultraviolet Radiation of Wavelengths between 180 nm and 400 nm (Incoherent Optical Radiation)." *Health Physics* 49, no. 2 (August), 331–340.

———— 1985b. "Guidelines on Limits of Exposure to Laser Radiation of Wavelengths between 180 nm and 1 nm." *Health Physics* 49, no. 2 (August), 341–359.

———— 1988. "Guidelines on Limits of Exposure to Radiofrequency Electromagnetic Fields in the Frequency Range from 100 kHz to 300 GHz." *Health Physics* 54, no. 1 (January), 115–123.

———— 1991. "Health Issues of Ultraviolet 'A' Sunbeds Used for Cosmetic Purposes." *Health Physics* 61, no. 2 (August), 285–288.

Johnson, D. W., and W. A. Goetz. 1985. *Patient Exposure Trends in Medical and Dental Radiography*. Rockville, Md.: Center for Devices and Radiological Health, U.S. Department of Health and Human Services.

Johnson, G. Timothy, ed. 1982. "Microwaves." *Harvard Medical School Health Letter* 7, no. 10 (August), 1–2 and 5.

Little, J. B. 1986. "Biological Effects of Low-Level Radiation Exposure." In *Radiology: Diagnosis—Imaging—Intervention,* vol. 1, ed. J. M. Taveras and J. T. Ferrucci. Philadelphia: J. P. Lippincott.

Mettler, F. A., Jr., M. Davis, C. A. Kelsey, R. Rosenberg, and A. Williams. 1987. "Analytical Modeling of Worldwide Medical Radiation Use." *Health Physics* 52, no. 2 (February), 133–141.

Mettler, F. A., Jr., W. K. Sinclair, L. Anspaugh, C. Edington, J. H. Harley, R. C. Ricks, P. B. Selby, E. W. Webster, and H. O. Wyckoff. 1990: "The 1986 and 1988 UNSCEAR Reports: Findings and Recommendations." *Health Physics* 58, no. 3 (March), 241–250.

Moeller, D. W., J. W. N. Hickey, and G. D. Schmidt. 1988. "Radiation from Consumer Products." *Consumers' Research* 71, no. 12 (December), 25–29.

Moore, Taylor. 1990. "Pursuing the Science of EMF." *EPRI Journal,* 15, no. 1 (January/February), 4–17.

Nair, I., M. G. Morgan, and H. K. Florig. 1989. *Biological Effects of Power Frequency Electric and Magnetic Fields*. Washington, D.C.: Office of Technology Assessment.

NCRP. 1987a. *Exposure of the Population in the United States and Canada from Natural Background Radiation*. Report no. 94. Bethesda, Md.

———— 1987b. *Ionizing Radiation Exposure of the Population of the United States*. Report no. 93. Bethesda, Md.

———— 1987c. *Radiation Exposure of the U.S. Population from Consumer Products and Miscellaneous Sources*. Report no. 95. Bethesda, Md.

———— 1989. *Exposure of the U.S. Population from Diagnostic Medical Radiation*. Report no. 100. Bethesda, Md.

NRC. 1990. *Population Dose Commitments due to Radioactive Releases from Nuclear Power Plant Sites in 1987*. Report NUREG/CR-2850, vol. 9. Washington, D.C.

———— 1991. *Information Digest, 1991 Edition*. Report NUREG-1350, vol. 3. Washington, D.C.: Office of the Controller.

Penna-Franca, E., M. Fiszman, N. Lobao, C. Costa-Ribeiro, H. Trindade, P. L. Dos Santos, and D. Batista. 1968. "Radioactivity in Brazil Nuts." *Health Physics* 14, no. 2 (February), 95–99.

Shepard, Michael. 1987. "EMF: The Debate on Health Effects." *EPRI Journal* 12, no. 7 (October/November), 4–15.

Shore, Roy E. (Department of Environmental Medicine, New York University). 1991. Private communication to author.

Tanner, Melissa. 1990. "Increasing Use, Power of Lasers Make Eye Protection Essential." *Occupational Health & Safety,* July, pp. 44–46.

U.S. Department of Health and Human Services. 1970. "Microwave Ovens: Performance Standards." Code of Federal Regulations, Title 42, Part 78.

10

Standards

Guidelines and recommendations for limiting exposures to a variety of occupational and environmental contaminants have been developed by many organizations. For example, the EPA, through its National Ambient Air Quality Standards, has established limits for airborne contaminants in the outdoor environment (Chapter 2). The EPA has also set standards for various contaminants in rivers and streams (Chapter 4). Guidelines for limiting exposures to chemical and physical stresses in the workplace have been developed by the American Conference of Governmental Industrial Hygienists (Chapter 3). Standards for environmental and occupational exposures to ionizing radiation have been set by the EPA, and the NRC and Occupational Safety and Health Administration have produced specific regulations for complying with them. Guidelines for protection against nonionizing radiation have been developed by the International Radiation Protection Association (Chapter 9).

In some cases both primary or basic and secondary standards have been established. Primary standards for air and water contaminants limit concentrations of contaminants with a view to protecting human health. In the case of air pollution, the secondary standards are designed to protect agricultural crops and property, such as buildings and statues; in the case of drinking water, secondary standards pertain to aesthetic aspects such as temperature, color, taste, and odor. Many of the secondary standards for contaminants in air and water are more stringent than the primary standards. In the case of protection against ionizing radiation, the secondary standards provide guides (for example, permissible concentrations of radioactive materials in air or water) that, if implemented, will assure compliance with the basic standards (the dose limits).

Many of the guidelines formulated by private organizations, such as the ACGIH, have also been incorporated in some form into federal, state, and local regulations. However, these regulations have a number of limitations, particularly in the adequacy and thoroughness of the underlying scientific data.

1. In only a very few instances have data been developed with a view to setting standards. Most data are by-products of descriptive and analytic studies designed to test specific scientific hypotheses (AAEE, 1983).
2. The data contain a range of uncertainties—not only those commonly encountered in the study of any biological system, but also uncertainties involved in extrapolating animal data to humans.
3. Few standards take into account all possible population groups. For example, most standards for workers are oriented to protecting adult males; they ignore the greater susceptibilities of pregnant women and other groups. Similarly, few standards take into account differences in weight, size, diet, and lifestyle among various population groups (for example, Japanese versus Americans). One way to overcome this problem would be to express the total intake limit on a given contaminant in terms of the allowable intake per unit of body weight.
4. Despite a consensus that standards for the general public should be much more stringent than those for workers, there is little coordination between the standards or among the agencies responsible for setting them. Moreover, there are no standards limiting concentrations of airborne contaminants inside dwellings and office buildings.
5. Some standards do not apply to all sources of a given contaminant. For example, guidelines for acceptable radiation doses to workers and the general public do not include exposures from natural background radiation and from medical applications.
6. Standards for the ambient environment and for protection of the public are commonly set for individual contaminants in individual environmental media—air, water, food, and soil—even though it is the total intake of the contaminant that is important.
7. In some instances, such as the case of exposures to magnetic and electric fields, there is a lack of definitive data or sound

epidemiologic evidence on which to base standards. Yet public pressure and the fact that exposures are occurring make standards necessary even when their basis is suspect. Too often, the public neither appreciates nor accepts the tentative nature of such standards.

8. Many standards, such as those for controlling airborne contaminants in the workplace or nonionizing radiation in the occupational and ambient environments, assume that there is a threshold for associated health effects, even though many public health experts believe that most environmental stresses have some impact however low the dose.

9. In most cases, the risks associated with exposures as expressed by the limits in various standards have not been quantified. Unless the risks are quantified, it is not possible to compare the stringency of, or the protection afforded by, standards that have been developed for different environmental contaminants or stresses.

10. Except in the case of air and water, few contaminant limits have been developed for protection of the natural environment, property, or aesthetic features. Similar considerations need to be applied to other environmental stresses.

11. Few standards consider the effects of exposures to a combination of occupational and environmental contaminants and stresses. In many cases, simultaneous exposure to two contaminants has synergistic effects; that is, the combination has a greater effect upon health than the sum of the two independent exposures.

12. Only the standards developed for radiation protection have established limits both for the exposure of individuals and for the number of people that should be permitted to be exposed at these levels (the collective population dose). A similar approach might be usefully applied to other occupational and environmental contaminants.

To provide insights that can be useful in developing standards for other kinds of exposures, this chapter reviews the current approach to setting standards for protection against ionizing radiation. One major accomplishment of these activities has been the establishment of a framework for coordinating radiation standards throughout the world.

Another has been the development of a risk-based approach to establishing associated dose limits. The resulting system permits comparison of partial and whole-body exposures on the basis of their relative health (morbidity and mortality) risks. These comparative data provide a scientific basis on which to set comparable limits, in terms of the associated risks, for exposures to the whole body and to individual organs.

Development of the Basis for Dose Limits

Shortly after the discovery of X rays in 1895 and of naturally occurring radioactive materials in 1896, reports of radiation injuries began to appear in the published literature. Recognizing the need for protection, physicists recommended limits on the allowable doses from X-ray generators. Their primary concern was to avoid direct physical symptoms. As early as 1902, however, scientists suggested that radiation exposures might also have latent effects, such as the development of cancer. This hypothesis was confirmed for external sources during the next two decades and for internally deposited radionuclides by 1930, when bone cancers were reported among workers using paint containing radium (Eisenbud, 1978).

As methods to control radiation were developed, and as people learned more about its potential long-term effects, reductions in dose limits were recommended. Initially, recommendations were developed on an informal basis. This changed in 1928 with the establishment of the International X-Ray and Radium Protection Committee (known today as the International Commission on Radiological Protection, ICRP) and the U.S. Advisory Committee on X-Ray and Radium Protection (known today as the National Council on Radiation Protection and Measurements, NCRP). The International Committee and its successor have provided a forum in which radiation protection experts from throughout the world can meet regularly, discuss the latest data on the biological effects of ionizing radiation, and formally propose radiation protection standards for application throughout the world. Today the ICRP and its scientific committees continue to formulate guidelines and recommendations on a wide range of occupational and environmental radiation protection matters. Since there are close ties between the NCRP and the ICRP, their recommendations tend to be in close conformity (Moeller, 1990).

In 1927 Hermann J. Muller's report on his experiments with *Drosophila* flies (Muller, 1927) aroused concern about possible genetic effects of radiation exposures in humans. This consideration shaped radiation protection guidelines and standards from the end of World War II until about 1960. During this same period, attention was focused on dose limits for occupational exposures. As public concern increased about worldwide exposures through fallout from atmospheric weapons tests, attention shifted to the need for dose limits for members of the public. In 1959 the Federal Radiation Council was created to provide federal policy on human radiation exposure and was charged with establishing dose limits for the public (Federal Radiation Council, 1960). At this same time, epidemiological studies showed an increase in leukemia among the survivors of the World War II nuclear bombings of Japan but failed to demonstrate the previously anticipated genetic effects. As a result, the focus gradually shifted from using genetic effects to using somatic effects, primarily leukemia, as the basis for the development of radiation protection standards. In 1970 the Committee on the Biological Effects of Ionizing Radiation reported that solid tumors (such as cancers of the lung, breast, bone, and thyroid), instead of leukemia, were the governing effects of human exposures to ionizing radiation (BEIR, 1972). As a result, the basis for the development of radiation standards shifted again and has remained primary ever since (BEIR, 1980, 1990).

In 1977 the ICRP broke new ground by proposing a mathematical system that would permit radiation protection standards to be based on what was considered to be an acceptable level of risk (ICRP, 1977). In 1987 the NCRP reinforced this effort with its *Recommendations on Limits for Exposure to Ionizing Radiation* (NCRP, 1987). In 1991 the ICRP further refined the risk-based approach (ICRP, 1991a). Included in this report were the findings that, owing to errors in earlier calculations of the doses received by the survivors of the nuclear bombings in Japan, the effects of radiation may be higher than previously stated (BEIR, 1990). The 1991 ICRP recommendations will undoubtedly serve as the basis for radiation protection standards for the next several decades. Table 10.1 summarizes this evolution of radiation protection standards.

Table 10.2 summarizes the ICRP recommendations for occupational whole-body external dose limits for the years 1934–1990. Many of these recommendations, and those of the NCRP, have been incor-

Table 10.1 Evolution of the basis for dose limits for ionizing radiation, 1900–1990

Approximate period	Protection criteria
1900–1930	Avoidance of immediate physical symptoms
1930–1950	Avoidance of longer-term biological symptoms, plus concern for genetic effects
1950–1960	Concern for genetic effects (and leukemia)
1960–1970	Concern for somatic effects (primarily leukemia)
1970–	Concern for somatic effects (primarily solid tumors)
1980–	Application of a risk-based approach to radiation protection standards
1990–	Expansion of risk approach to include additional effects, such as loss in life expectancy and effects of morbidity

Table 10.2 ICRP recommendations for occupational whole-body equivalent dose limits, 1934–1990

	Dose limit		
Year	Per day	Per week	Per year
1934	0.2 roentgen		72 roentgens
1950		0.3 roentgen	
1958		0.1 rem	5 (N − 18) rem[a]
1965			5 rem (maximum)
1977			50 mSv (5 rem); based on acceptable risk[b]
1990			50 mSv (5 rem); maximum of 100 mSv (10 rem) in any 5 years

a. Where N is the age of the worker receiving the exposure.
b. Recommended that the average dose to all workers not exceed 10% of the limit for individual workers.

porated into NRC regulations (NRC, 1991). As the table shows, the ICRP currently recommends a dose-rate limit of 50 mSv per year; however, no individual worker should receive more than 100 mSv over any 5-year period. This allowance is comparable to the NCRP's recommendation that the occupational dose never exceed 10 mSv times a worker's age (NCRP, 1987): under either system, a worker who was first exposed to ionizing radiation at age 20 would be permitted to have accumulated 0.4 Sv by age 40.

Over the years there have been significant reductions in the levels of occupational radiation exposure considered acceptable (Figure 10.1). However, except in the very early years, these reductions have occurred as a result not of observed health effects but of improved control technology and better understanding of the risks associated with radiation exposures.

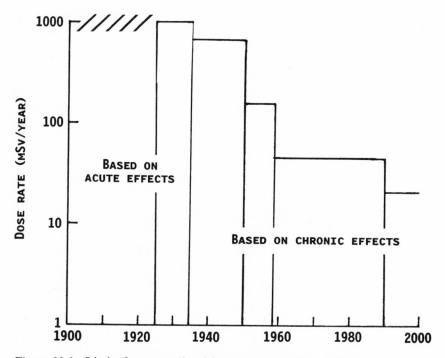

Figure 10.1 Limits for occupational exposures to ionizing radiation, 1900–1990. The limits since 1925 are based on recommendations of the ICRP and its predecessors.

Current Standards

The current system of radiation protection is based on the following general principles (ICRP, 1991a):

The practice must be justified; that is, it must have a positive net benefit.

The practice must be optimized; that is, all exposures must be kept as low as reasonably achievable, with economic and social factors taken into account.

Doses to individuals must not exceed established limits.

Occupational Dose Limits

Table 10.3, column 2, summarizes the current recommended dose limits for radiation workers. Three important features of these recommendations are:

Dose limits are provided for short-term (1-year) as well as for longer-term (5-year) exposures.

Dose limits apply to the sums of the doses received from both external and internal exposures.

The standards are specified in terms of the effective dose, a unit that expresses partial-body doses in terms of equivalent doses to the whole body. This approach permits the addition, on an equivalent-risk basis, of partial and whole-body doses.

Dose Limits for the General Public

Dose limits for the general public are set lower than those for radiation workers for a variety of reasons (NCRP, 1971):

The population includes pregnant women, infants and children, the sick, and the elderly, each of whom may represent a group at increased risk; for example, their metabolism and breathing rates may be different from those of an adult radiation worker.

Members of the public may be exposed 24 hours a day, 7 days a week, for their entire lifetime, whereas exposures of workers are generally limited to their working (adult) lifetime and presumably only to the time they are on the job.

In the case of most environmental sources, members of the public

Table 10.3 Occupational and population dose limits

| | Radiation worker | General population | |
		Individuals	Total population
Annual limit	50 mSv	5 mSv	
Cumulative limit	20 mSv per year averaged over any 5 years	1 mSv per year, averaged over any 5 consecutive years	≪ 1 mSv per year
Relative magnitude	100%	5%	≪ 5%

have had no choice about whether they would be exposed, and they may receive no direct benefit from the exposure.

Many members of the public are already being exposed to risks in their own occupations; those who are radiation workers may already be receiving significant exposures on the job.

Members of the public are not subject to the selection, supervision, and monitoring afforded radiation workers.

Even when individual doses are sufficiently low that the risk to the individual is extremely small, the collective risk in the population may justify additional limits on exposures.

Current radiation dose limits recommended for the general population are summarized in Table 10.3, columns 3 and 4. Although the NCRP would permit members of the public to receive up to 5 mSv in a single year, it concurs with the ICRP that over the longer term the whole-body dose rate should not exceed 1 mSv per year, or 5 percent of the cumulative dose-rate limit for radiation workers (NCRP, 1987; ICRP, 1991a). The average annual dose to the population as a whole is expected to be well below these values except in the unlikely event of a major nuclear accident.

The Concept of the Effective Dose

The ICRP has used the concept of the effective dose to develop a system that provides a unit useful in expressing radiation protection standards for both whole-body and partial-body exposures on an equal-risk basis (ICRP, 1977, 1991a). One of the benefits of this concept is that it permits internal exposures to be converted to equivalent whole-body doses and to be summed with external exposures to calculate total dose. In developing this system the ICRP (1) based the limits on the total risk (both mortality and morbidity) to all tissues and on genetic effects in the first two generations of offspring; and (2) considered, in the case of internally deposited radionuclides, not only the dose occurring during the year of intake but also the dose resulting from the continuing presence of this material in the body. This is referred to as the committed dose, and a time limit of 50 years has been selected for its assessment.

Parameters that must be taken into account in developing this system include the probability that radiation will induce a given type of cancer or genetic effect, the probability that the cancer or effect will be lethal (the cancer lethality fraction), the years of life that will be lost as a result of the death, and the associated health care and psychological impacts. These parameters are then used to calculate the contributions to the total risk that result from exposures to individual body organs (the tissue-weighting factors). These factors provide a numerical basis on which the dose to a single organ or tissue can be weighted to estimate the equivalent whole-body (effective) dose.

Calculation of Risk of Death from Exposures to Individual Organs

On the basis of epidemiological and biological studies, the risk of a cancer fatality (the fatal cancer probability coefficient) can be estimated for given levels of dose to various organs. Basic to this calculation is the concept of collective dose, a unit developed to express the integrated dose to a given population group. For example, if 10,000 people each received an average whole-body dose of 1 Sv, the collective dose would be 10,000 person-Sv (1 million person-rem). Similarly, if 20,000 people each received an average dose of 0.5 Sv, or if 5,000 each received an average dose of 2 Sv, the integrated or total population dose would be 10,000 person-Sv.

Although the concept of collective dose is useful in evaluating the public health impacts of radiation exposures, it should be applied only if it can be assumed that:

   there is a linear relationship between the dose and its resulting biological effects the potential effects of the rate at which the doses are received (and whether they are fractionated or protracted) are not important

the individual doses and dose rates are sufficiently low that only stochastic (latent) effects need be considered

the doses are sufficiently high to be statistically significant

Thus, the concept of collective dose is not applicable if the doses to individuals in the target population group are either very high or very low. For example, if 1,000 people each received 10 Sv the collective dose would be 10,000 person-Sv. Yet such a dose, received over a short period, would be fatal to all members of the exposed group. At the other extreme, if 1 billion people each received 10 microsievert (1 mrem), the collective dose would likewise be 10,000 person-Sv; however, it would be next to impossible to demonstrate any excess ill effects among the exposed group.

The following examples show how epidemiological data and the concept of collective dose can be used to estimate the number of excess deaths (the fatal cancer probability coefficient) in a population group that has received a known equivalent dose to an individual organ or tissue.

Lung Cancer

Studies of uranium miners and the survivors of the nuclear bombings in Japan indicate that for each 10,000 person-Sv of collective dose to the lungs of a given population group, there will be an excess of about 90 lung cancers; that is, about 90 people will develop lung cancer who would not otherwise have done so. Medical experience has shown that about 95 percent of the lung cancers induced by ionizing radiation are fatal. This is referred to as the cancer lethality fraction (see Table 10.4, column 2). On this basis, one can estimate the risk of death from cancer as a result of radiation exposures to the lungs to be:

$$\frac{90 \text{ excess cancers}}{10,000 \text{ person-Sv}} \times (0.95 \text{ fatality rate})$$

$$= 85 \times 10^{-4}/\text{Sv}.$$

This number has been designated by the ICRP (1991a) as the fatal cancer probability coefficient for lung cancer (see Table 10.4, column 3).

Table 10.4   Fatal cancer and adjusted probability coefficients, tissue-weighting factors, and annual occupational dose limits for individual tissues and organs

Tissue or organ	Cancer lethality fraction	Fatal cancer probability coefficient $(10^{-4}/Sv)$	Adjusted probability coefficient $(10^{-4}/Sv)$	Tissue-weighting factor (w_T)[a]	Annual equivalent dose limit (mSv)
Gonads	—	—	133	0.20[b]	100
Ovary	0.70	10	15		
Bone marrow	0.99	50	104	0.12	150
Colon	0.55	85	103	0.12	150
Lung	0.95	85	80	0.12	150
Stomach	0.90	110	100	0.12	150
Bladder	0.50	30	29	0.05	400
Breast	0.50	20	36	0.05	400
Liver	0.95	15	16	0.05	400
Esophagus	0.95	30	24	0.05	400
Thyroid	0.10	8	15	0.05	400
Bone surface	0.70	5	7	0.01	500[c]
Skin	0.002	2	4	0.01	500[c]
Remainder[d]	0.80	50	59	0.05	400
Total		500	725	1.00	

a. To avoid implications of accuracy beyond what the biological data will justify, the tissue-weighting factors for the various tissues and organs have been assigned one of four values: 0.01, 0.05, 0.12, or 0.20.
b. Total for the gonads (including cancer in the ovaries).
c. Based on deterministic effects.
d. The equivalent dose for the remaining body organs is the estimated mean equivalent dose over the whole body excluding the specified tissues and organs.

Bone Marrow (Leukemia)

Studies since World War II of the survivors of the nuclear bombings in Japan indicate that if 10,000 people have received a dose of 1 Sv (a collective dose of 10,000 person-Sv) to their red bone marrow, after a latency period about 50 excess cases of leukemia will develop in this group. Assuming that 99 percent of these cases are fatal, one can estimate the risk of death (fatal cancer probability coefficient) from leukemia as a result of exposures to the bone marrow to be (ICRP, 1991a):

$$\frac{50 \text{ excess cancers}}{10,000 \text{ person-Sv}} \times (0.99 \text{ fatality rate})$$

$$= 50 \times 10^{-4}/\text{Sv}.$$

Breast Cancer

Epidemiological data indicate that radiation exposures of the breast produce an excess of about 80 breast cancers per 10,000 person-Sv. Assuming that breast cancer is fatal 50 percent of the time, and assuming that the population being exposed consists of 50 percent men and 50 percent women, one can estimate the fatal cancer probability coefficient from exposures of the female breasts to be (ICRP, 1991a):

$$\frac{80 \text{ excess cancers}}{10,000 \text{ person-Sv}} \times (0.5 \text{ fatality rate})$$

$$\times (0.5 \text{ of population})$$

$$= 20 \times 10^{-4}/\text{Sv}.$$

Thyroid Cancer

Data indicate that radiation exposures of the thyroid produce an excess of about 80 thyroid cancers per 10,000 person-Sv. Assuming a fatality rate of 10 percent for thyroid cancer, one can estimate the fatal cancer probability coefficient to be (ICRP, 1991a):

$$\frac{80 \text{ excess cancers}}{10,000 \text{ person-Sv}} \times (0.10 \text{ fatality rate})$$

$$= 8 \times 10^{-4}/\text{Sv}.$$

Similar calculations can be made to estimate the excess deaths resulting from exposures of other body organs, including deaths due to cancers of the reproductive organs. These data are summarized in Table 10.4, column 3. The sum of all the fatal cancer probability coefficients for radiation-induced cancers in all body tissues and organs is 500×10^{-4}/Sv, the value currently being used in radiation protection analyses and risk assessments.

Calculation of Adjusted Probability Coefficients

Recognizing that radiation-induced cancers have effects besides mortality, the ICRP has adjusted the fatal cancer probability coefficients to take into account not only the death itself but also the other mortality effects (as reflected by the years of productive life lost) among individuals who died, as well as the morbidity effects of the cancers that were not fatal (as reflected in the reduced quality of life for the victim, associated health care costs, and emotional impacts on family and friends) (ICRP, 1985, 1991a). In making this adjustment, the increase in the fatal cancer probability coefficient for a cancer that is difficult to cure, and thus has a high cancer lethality fraction, is less than that for a cancer that is less fatal. Similarly, the increase in the fatal cancer probability coefficient is less for a cancer that results in fewer years of productive life lost (Table 10.5). The following examples show the techniques used in making these adjustments. Cancers of the lung and thyroid illustrate the adjustments for a cancer that is difficult to cure and one that has a low probability of causing death.

Lung Cancer

Given that the percentage of lung cancers considered to be lethal— that is, the cancer lethality fraction—is 95 percent (Table 4, column 2), 5 percent are assumed not to be lethal. The fatal cancer probability coefficient for lung cancer (calculated earlier) is 85×10^{-4}/Sv. The adjusted probability coefficient is the product of the fatal cancer probability coefficient times one plus the percentage of lung cancers that are not fatal (0.05), multiplied by a factor of 0.9 to account for the years of life lost (see Table 10.5, column 3):

$$\{(85 \times 10^{-4}/\text{Sv})\,(1.00 + 0.05)\}\,\{0.9\}$$
$$= 80 \times 10^{-4}/\text{Sv}.$$

In this case the adjustment in the fatal cancer probability coefficient is relatively small.

Table 10.5   Years of life lost and adjustment factors for various cancers induced by ionizing radiation

Type of cancer	Years of life lost	Adjustment factor
Bladder	9.8	0.65
Bone marrow	30.9	2.06
Bone surface	15.0	1.00
Breast	18.2	1.21
Colon	12.5	0.83
Esophagus	11.5	0.77
Gonads	20.0	1.33
Liver	15.0	1.00
Lung	13.5	0.90
Ovary	16.8	1.12
Skin	15.0	1.00
Stomach	12.4	0.83
Thyroid	15.0	1.00
Remainder	13.7	0.91

Thyroid Cancer

Because 10 percent of thyroid cancers are considered to be lethal, 90 percent are considered not to be lethal. The fatal cancer probability coefficient for thyroid cancers is $8 \times 10^{-4}/Sv$. The adjusted probability coefficient is therefore the product of the fatal cancer probability coefficient times one plus the percentage of thyroid cancers that are not fatal (0.90), multiplied by a factor of 1.0 to account for the years of life lost (see Table 10.5, column 3):

$$\{(8 \times 10^{-4}/Sv) (1.00 \times 0.90)\}\{1.00\}$$

$$= 15.2 \times 10^{-4}/Sv.$$

In this case the adjustment in the fatal cancer probability coefficient is relatively large.

Adjusted probability coefficients for cancers of the other organs can be calculated in the same way. These values are recorded in Table 10.4, column 4.

Calculation of Tissue-Weighting Factors (w_T)

As column 4 of Table 10.4 shows, the sum of the adjusted probability coefficients for all types of cancers in all organs of the body, plus the associated hereditary effects, is about 725×10^{-4}/Sv. This value can be used to calculate tissue-weighting factors, which in turn can be used to estimate the dose limits for exposures to individual organs.

As calculated above, the adjusted probability coefficient for lung cancer is 80×10^{-4}/Sv. Therefore, cancer of the lungs represents 80/725, or about 12 percent, of the sum of all the adjusted probability coefficients. In other words, if the entire body were exposed to ionizing radiation, the risk and consequences of developing lung cancer would represent about 12 percent of the total risk arising through the development of cancers in other organs and through the production of hereditary effects. This value, 0.12, is called the tissue-weighting factor (w_t) for the lungs. Similarly, the adjusted probability coefficient for thyroid cancer is 15×10^{-4}/Sv. Therefore, thyroid cancer represents 15/725, or 2 percent, of the sum of all the adjusted probability coefficients. Because differences in the values calculated by this approach would imply far more accuracy than is justified by the biological data, the ICRP has recommended that tissue-weighting factors for the various organs be assigned one of four values: 0.01, 0.05, 0.12, and 0.20. The value assigned to the thyroid is 0.05. Tissue-weighting factors for all organs are listed in Table 10.4, column 5.

Calculation of Dose Limits for Individual Organs

The tissue-weighting factors can be used to calculate the effective dose (whole-body equivalent dose) for partial-body exposures. This process, in turn, can be used to set dose-rate limits for individual organs that are comparable (in terms of risk) to the dose-rate limits for the whole body. For example, the tissue-weighting factor for the lungs is 0.12; that is, the morbidity and mortality resulting from excess lung cancer induced by radiation represent one-eighth (12 percent) of the total risk associated with whole-body exposures to ionizing radiation. Since the longer-term ICRP dose-rate limit for the whole body is 20 mSv per year, the equivalent dose-rate limit for the lungs (assuming this is the only portion of the body being exposed) would be eight times as high. That is, the dose rate for the lungs that is equivalent to 20 mSv per year to the whole body is:

$$\frac{20\ \text{mSv}}{0.12} \sim 150\ \text{mSv per year.}$$

A similar annual limit would apply to the red bone marrow, colon, and stomach.

Likewise, the dose rate for the thyroid that is comparable to 20 mSv per year to the whole body would be:

$$\frac{20\ \text{mSv}}{0.05} = 400\ \text{mSv per year.}$$

A similar annual limit would apply to the bladder, breast, liver, esophagus, and "remainder" organs.

By this same approach, the dose-rate limit for the skin and bone surfaces would be:

$$\frac{20\ \text{mSv}}{0.01} = 2,000\ \text{mSv per year.}$$

Because this is an unacceptably high dose rate, and because the technology for reducing the rate to values well below this number is readily available, the ICRP has based the limit for the skin and bone surfaces on deterministic effects—that is, effects that have a dose threshold for occurrence. To avoid deterministic effects, the ICRP recommends that the lifetime dose to any body organ for a radiation worker be limited to no more than 20 Sv. For a 40-year working lifetime, the dose would amount to 500 mSv per year. On this basis, the ICRP has selected an annual dose limit of 500 mSv for the skin and bone surface.

Annual equivalent dose limits for a full range of body organs calculated on the basis of the tissue-weighting factors developed by the ICRP are listed in column 6 of Table 10.4. These limits are illustrative only. Although many radionuclides preferentially deposit in single or-

gans (for example, radioactive iodine in the thyroid; radioactive strontium, radium, and plutonium in the bone; and airborne radioactive
materials in the lungs), these materials may also cause radiation exposures to tissues adjacent to these organs. In addition, soluble radionuclides that are inhaled (and initially cause exposure solely to the lungs)
may subsequently be taken up by the blood and deposited in other
organs. Calculations of annual limits on intake for individual radionuclides (see below) must assess the doses to all portions of the body
and keep the intake limit low enough that the combined fractional
doses to the several affected organs do not exceed the effective dose-
rate limit (20 mSv per year).

Assessment of Internal Exposures

In the case of external radiation sources, particularly those that cause
whole-body exposures, compliance with dose limits can be assessed
through radiation surveys, personnel monitoring, or both. These evaluations are not possible in the case of doses resulting from the intake
of radionuclides into the body. Instead, secondary or derived limits
must be developed that will assure that the basic dose limits are being
observed. The following sections describe the basis for the derivation
of two of these secondary limits.

Annual Limits on Intake and Derived Air Concentrations

The annual limit on intake (ALI) is the quantity of a given radionuclide
that, if ingested or inhaled, will result in an uptake in the body that
will yield a committed dose to the affected organs over the subsequent
50-year period that is equivalent to the effective dose limit (ICRP,
1991a, 1991b). If a radionuclide causes exposure of the total body, the
applicable annual dose limit will be 20 mSv. If a radionuclide causes
exposure to only a single organ, the dose-rate limit for that organ will
be as indicated in Table 10.4. If the radionuclide causes exposure to
several body organs, the sum of the fractions obtained by dividing the
dose to each of the affected organs by the dose limit for that organ
must not exceed one.

Estimates of ALIs require information about several factors. If the
material is being inhaled, these include the deposition, retention, and

uptake of the radionuclide in the lungs (which depends on particle size and solubility) and the breathing patterns of the exposed worker (through the nose or mouth and the rate of breathing). If the material is being ingested, these factors include whether it is soluble and will be taken up by the blood and preferentially deposited in one or more organs. If the material is insoluble, the major concern will be exposure of the gastrointestinal tract as the material moves through the body. Other considerations include the efficiency of transfer of the radionuclide to the bloodstream, the movement and efficiency of the radionuclide's deposition in the body, the mass(es) of the organ(s) in which the radionuclide deposits, the length of time it remains there, and the annual equivalent-dose limit(s) for the portion(s) of the body affected. It is also necessary to know the quantity of radionuclide ingested or inhaled, its physical half-life, the types and energies of the radiations it emits, and the associated radiation weighting factors. Combining this and other information, one can estimate the quantity of the given radionuclide that, if ingested or inhaled, would yield a committed dose that is equal to the respective annual dose limit for the portion(s) of the body affected. This quantity is the annual limit on intake. Table 10.6 lists ALIs for inhalation and ingestion for some of the more common radionuclides.

If the major avenue of intake is inhalation, an estimate can be made of the derived air concentration (DAC) for the given radionuclide, taking into account the hours of exposure per year and the breathing rate. For example, the DAC for occupational exposure to any radionuclide is the concentration in air that, if breathed by an adult for an assumed occupational exposure time of 2,000 hours per year, will result in the ALI via inhalation. Numerically, the DAC can be calculated as follows:

$$DAC = \frac{ALI}{(2,000 \text{ hr./yr.}) (60 \text{ min./hr.}) (20,000 \text{ cm}^3/\text{min.})}$$

The Committed Dose

Once a radionuclide has been deposited in the body, the exposed person is "committed" to the dose resulting from the decay of that radionuclide as long as it is present in the body. For radionuclides with effective half-lives of only a few months (that is, those that have

Table 10.6 Annual limits on intake for occupational exposures to radionuclides

| | Most restrictive limit on annual intake[a] | | | |
| | Inhalation | | Ingestion | |
Radionuclide	Bq	μCi	Bq	μCi
Hydrogen-3[b]	1×10^9	3×10^4	1×10^9	3×10^4
Carbon-14[c]	4×10^7	1×10^3	4×10^7	1×10^3
Phosphorus-32	5×10^6	1.5×10^2	8×10^6	2×10^2
Sulfur-35	3×10^7	8×10^2	7×10^7	1.5×10^3
Cobalt-60	4×10^5	10	3×10^6	80
Strontium-90	6×10^4	1.5	6×10^5	15
Iodine-131	1×10^6	25	8×10^5	20
Cesium-137	2×10^6	50	1×10^6	25
Radium-226	9×10^3	0.25	9×10^4	2.5
Plutonium-239	3×10^2	8×10^{-3}	4×10^4	1

a. Since absorption through the lungs frequently differs from that through the GI tract, intake limits for inhalation frequently differ from those for ingestion. Intake limits also vary with the chemical compound in which the radionuclide is incorporated. The values shown here are those for the most readily absorbed compounds.

b. As vapor.

c. As an organic compound.

a short radioactive half-life or are rapidly excreted), the committed dose is delivered, in the main, during the year following intake. For radionuclides with long effective half-lives (that is, those that have a long radioactive half-life and are retained a long time in the body), only a fraction of the total dose will be delivered to the body during the year in which the radionuclide was initially inhaled or ingested. In fact, for radionuclides with very long effective half-lives, neither the total dose nor a full expression of the associated risk can be expected to be manifested during the lifetime of the worker. Consequently, the committed dose from the lifelong intake of some radionuclides with long effective half-lives may overestimate, by a factor of two or more, the actual lifetime risk. As a result, care must be taken in using such data for epidemiological studies.

The NCRP (1987) recommends that use of the committed dose associated with the intake of a given radionuclide be restricted to radiation protection planning, such as in the design of facilities and the development of manufacturing processes and research protocols; to the demonstration of compliance with those plans; and to the calculation of ALIs and DACs. In the opinion of the NCRP, the committed dose does not in itself constitute a sufficient basis for evaluation of the potential health effects of radiation exposures in individuals; rather, such evaluations should be based on estimates of the actual absorbed dose being delivered to the tissues and organs in question.

The General Outlook

The system that has been designed for developing recommendations for dose limits and standards for exposures to ionizing radiation has many desirable characteristics. The standards are based on associated risks to health; a procedure has been developed for expressing dose rates from internal and external exposures on the basis of their relative risks; there is a systematic relationship between limits for the general population and those for radiation workers; and, through the ICRP, the approach to these problems is uniform worldwide. These features might also prove useful in the development of permissible limits for exposures to other occupational and environmental stresses. For example, similar relationships might be developed and applied in setting limits for airborne concentrations of certain toxic chemicals in the workplace and the general environment.

Even this advanced system, however, has deficiencies. One of the most significant is that the given dose limits do not include exposures from natural radiation sources and the use of radiation in medicine and dentistry. In addition, the procedures used for calculating the annual limits on intake and the associated derived air concentrations are based on the assumption that the given radionuclide is the sole source of exposure to the person being exposed. If an individual is exposed to several radionuclides (as many members of the public are), suitable reductions must be made in the allowable intake limits. Nor does the existing system take into account that radionuclides released into outdoor air and water undergo chemical and physical changes as they move through various environmental chains. In the case of airborne releases, the particle size distribution and chemical composition

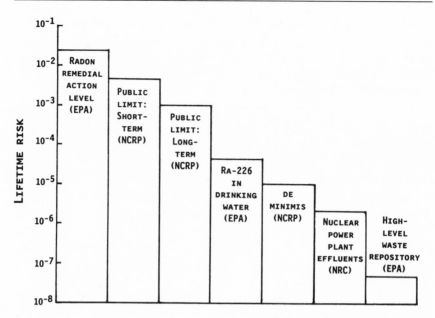

Figure 10.2   U.S. standards for exposures to various sources of ionizing radiation.

of the individual radionuclides will change. There will also be seasonal variations in the movement and behavior of individual radionuclides in the environment.

Another major deficiency lies in the inconsistent manner in which the system is being implemented. A review of the standards established in the United States for various radiation sources has found orders-of-magnitude differences in the lifetime risks associated with the currently permissible limits for exposures to technologically enhanced naturally occurring radiation sources (such as indoor radon), for short- and long-term exposures of population groups to artificial sources, for exposures resulting from liquid and airborne releases to the environment from nuclear power plants, and for potential exposures from the operation of the proposed deep geologic repository for the disposal of high-level radioactive wastes (Kocher, 1988) (Figure 10.2).

As studies of the effects of ionizing radiation produce more information, dose limits will undoubtedly be refined further. Such changes can be anticipated for all environmental contaminants. One fundamental problem that should be addressed in the meantime is the common public misconception that standards assure risk-free conditions. The public should be involved in the standards-setting process so that they will understand both the goals being sought and the means by which they are to be achieved. Experience has shown that, although the public will voluntarily accept risks, they will balk at accepting involuntary risks, particularly if they conclude that the risks are being imposed on them without full disclosure. The development and promulgation of standards must involve effective and continuing communication between the scientific community and the public at large (AAEE, 1983).

REFERENCES

AAEE. 1983. *Proceedings of the Seminar on Development and Assessment of Environmental Standards.* Annapolis, Md.
ACGIH. 1990. *1990–1991 Threshold Limit Values for Chemical Substances and Physical Agents and Biological Exposure Indices.* Cincinnati.
BEIR. 1972. *The Effects on Populations of Exposure to Low Levels of Ionizing Radiation.* Report no. I. Washington, D.C.: National Academy Press.
———— 1980. *The Effects on Populations of Exposure to Low Levels of Ionizing Radiation.* Report no. III. Washington, D.C.: National Academy Press.
———— 1990. *The Effects on Populations of Exposure to Low Levels of Ionizing Radiation.* Report no. V. Washington, D.C.: National Academy Press.
Eisenbud, M. 1978. *Environment, Technology, and Health: Human Ecology in Historical Perspective.* New York: New York University Press.
Federal Radiation Council. 1960. *Background Material for the Development of Radiation Protection Standards.* Report no. 1. Washington, D.C.: U.S. Department of Health, Education and Welfare.
ICRP. 1977. *Recommendations of the International Commission on Radiological Protection.* Publication 26, Annals of the ICRP, vol. 1, no. 3. New York: Pergamon Press.
———— 1985. *Quantitative Basis for Developing a Unified Index of Harm.* Publication 45, Annals of the ICRP, vol. 15, no. 3. New York: Pergamon Press.
———— 1991a. *1990 Recommendations of the International Commission on*

Radiological Protection. Publication 60, Annals of the ICRP, vol. 21, no. 1–3. New York: Pergamon Press.

———— 1991b. *Annual Limits on Intake of Radionuclides by Workers Based on the 1990 Recommendations.* Publication 61, Annals of the ICRP, vol. 21, no. 4. New York: Pergamon Press.

Kocher, D. C. 1988. "Review of Radiation Protection and Environmental Radiation Standards for the Public." *Nuclear Safety* 29, no. 4 (October–December), 463–475.

Moeller, Dade W. 1990. "History and Perspective on the Development of Radiation Protection Standards." In *Radiation Protection Today: The NCRP at Sixty Years.* Proceedings no. 11. Bethesda, Md.: National Council on Radiation Protection and Measurements.

Muller, Hermann J. 1927. "Artificial Transmutation of the Gene." *Science* 66, no. 1699 (11 July), 84–87.

NCRP, 1971. *Basic Radiation Protection Criteria.* Report no. 39. Bethesda, Md.

———— 1987. *Recommendations on Limits for Exposure to Ionizing Radiation.* Report no. 91. Bethesda, Md.

NRC. 1991. "Standards for Protection against Radiation." Code of Federal Regulations, Title 10, Part 20.

11

Monitoring

An environmental monitoring program has two basic objectives: to estimate exposures to people resulting from certain physical stresses (such as noise and radiation) and from toxic materials that are being, or have been, released and are subsequently being ingested or inhaled, and to determine whether the resulting exposures comply with the limits prescribed by regulations. Monitoring physical stresses may simply involve identifying the sources and measuring the magnitude of the stress. Monitoring releases of toxic materials involves much more. For airborne or waterborne releases, the first step will probably be to measure discharges at the sources, such as installations operated by industrial organizations, municipalities, state or federal governmental agencies, or nonprofit or other groups. Additional steps include assessing the movement or transport of specific contaminants within given environmental media (air, water, and soil), their transfer from one medium to another, and their chemical and biological transformation as they move within the environment. Data on exposures can, in turn, be used to estimate the doses to people. Data on the distribution of energies of physical stresses can be used to estimate the accompanying dose as a function of tissue depth and specific body organ. Data on the physical and chemical nature of toxic substances can be used to estimate their deposition and uptake by the body as well as the dose to various organs. Because there are so many avenues by which contaminants can cause exposures of people, most environmental monitoring specialists try to identify and trace the movement and behavior of several key contaminants through several environmental pathways. As a supplement to these measurements, they may also analyze the concentrations of selected contaminants in various ecological indicators, such as muds and biota from streams. Data on contaminants as a function of depth in muds can provide information on the history of contaminants in a stream; data on contaminants biologically concentrated in biota can provide information on contaminants whose concentrations in the stream itself are below the limits of analytic sensitivity.

Sampling and monitoring the environment are complex processes. In monitoring for physical stresses, such as electric and magnetic fields, the mere presence of people and their monitoring equipment may alter the environment in such a way as to make accurate measurements difficult. In addition, the position and location of the people being exposed (for example, whether they are standing on the ground, or near a tree or sitting inside an automobile) can alter the type and extent of the exposures they receive. In sampling to collect data on the health effects of airborne contaminants, the presence of both particles and gases is important, since they behave differently. For example, the size of airborne particles will significantly affect whether and where they will be deposited in the respiratory tract, and their chemical composition will determine where and how they move within the body and their potential effects on health. It is also important to know what other chemicals are associated with a given contaminant, since certain combinations of contaminants are synergistic; that is, the combination may have a more detrimental effect on health than the sum of the effects of the contaminants independently. For example, sulfur dioxide, a ubiquitous acidic gas that is highly soluble and is ordinarily entirely taken up in the throat and upper airways, where its effects on health are minimal, acutely impairs the functioning of the lungs when carried to the alveoli as an acid condensed on the surfaces of small particles (less than 5 micrometers in diameter).

Today many environmental monitoring programs have broader objectives than simply assessing the exposures and resulting doses to people. With worldwide concern about destruction of the ozone layer (which protects humans from excessive ultraviolet radiation), potential warming of the earth (the "greenhouse effect") as a result of releases of carbon dioxide, and acidic deposition as a result of releases of nitrogen and sulfur oxides, there is increasing interest in monitoring programs designed to assess both the quantities and trends in the discharges of pollutants that cause these effects.

Most environmental monitoring programs include an array of secondary objectives, such as predicting trends in exposures with time, determining critical pathway parameters, meeting legal requirements, and providing public information. They should also be designed so that they can be expanded for collecting data to evaluate exposures and doses associated with nonroutine releases that might occur as a result of an accident or some other emergency situation. Table 11.1 summarizes the types and purposes of environmental monitoring programs.

As a general rule, local environmental monitoring programs for industrial facilities are handled by plant personnel or environmental service contractors, whereas regional surveillance is handled by state and local environmental health and regulatory authorities. Close coordination between the facility operator and the local agencies is necessary if all objectives of the monitoring program are to be met. A well-planned program will usually involve some overlap in the activities of the several monitoring groups, including exchanges of samples and cross-checking of data.

Measuring Releases and Exposures

In assessing exposures to chemical contaminants, the first step should be to measure their concentrations in liquid and airborne effluents as they leave the facility. Air and water are the principal pathways both for direct exposures (through inhalation and the consumption of drinking water) and for the transport of contaminants from the point of release to other environmental media (such as milk and food). Measurements of airborne and waterborne contaminants leaving a plant can also provide advance information on impending problems in other environmental media. Since critical contaminants can be missed if only the obvious and easily measured effluents are monitored, or if monitoring ceases during key periods such as shutdowns for repairs and maintenance, such measurements should be made during the entire cycle of plant operations. Where measurements show releases to be minimal, using data based on environmental measurements to estimate population exposures may be difficult. In these cases it may be necessary to use data on the quantities and concentrations of the various contaminants in releases from the plant as input to computer models developed for estimating population exposures. Even so, some data should always be collected on environmental samples if for no other reason than to validate the computer model estimates.

Air samplers should be located in places where airborne concentrations and ground deposition of various contaminants are most likely to lead to human exposures. The selection of specific sampling sites should be based on the best available meteorological information, coupled with data on local land use. For rivers and streams, the primary sampling stations should be located above and below the target facility and at the intake of the first downstream water user. It is also advisable to sample nearby groundwater used as a source of drinking water.

Table 11.1 Types and purposes of environmental monitoring programs

Type of program	Purpose
Based on nature of the stress	
Physical stress	To assess the impact of environmental stresses such as noise and radiation, where the evaluation is based primarily on exposure measurements made in the field, not on samples collected and returned to the laboratory for analysis
Chemical stress	To assess exposures resulting from the ingestion and inhalation of chemical and radioactive contaminants
Based on geographic (spatial) coverage	
Local	To evaluate the impact of a single facility on the neighboring area
Regional	To evaluate the combined impact of emissions from several facilities on a larger area
Global	To determine worldwide impacts and trends, such as acidic deposition, depletion of the ozone layer, and the potential for global warming
Based on temporal considerations	
Preoperational	To determine potential contamination levels in the environment prior to operation of a new industrial facility; to train staff; to confirm the operation of laboratory and field equipment
Operational	To provide data on releases; to confirm adequacy of pollution controls
Postoperational	To assure proper site cleanup and restoration

Table 11.1   (continued)

Type of program	Purpose
Based on monitoring objectives	
Source related	To determine population exposures from a single source
Person related	To determine the total exposure to people from all sources
Environment related	To determine the impacts of several sources on features of the environment such as plants, trees, buildings, statues, soil, and water
Research related	To determine the transfer of specific pollutants from one environmental medium to another and to assess their chemical and biological transformation as they move within the environment; to determine ecological indicators of pollution; to confirm that the critical population group has been correctly identified and that the models being applied are accurate representations of the environment being monitored
Based on administrative and legal requirements	
Compliance related	To determine compliance with applicable regulations
Public information	To provide data and information for purposes of public relations

Measurements to determine exposures from physical stresses such as noise and ionizing and nonionizing radiation must often be made on a real-time basis. This is generally accomplished through the use of instruments placed near the people being exposed or in concentric rings at various distances from the source.

Table 11.2 summarizes the advantages and disadvantages of various sampling methods for the principal types of environmental contaminants and receptor media.

Designing a Program

Most environmental monitoring programs have at least four stages: collecting background data, collecting and analyzing samples, establishing temporal relationships, and assuring the validity of results.

Although the design depends to a major extent on the purposes of the program, the following discussion, which focuses on assessing exposures from a nuclear facility, generally applies to all monitoring programs. Table 11.3 lists representative sources of information on the development of monitoring programs for nuclear facilities.

Although a nuclear facility can be a source of direct external exposure to nearby population groups, inhalation and ingestion of radioactive materials released into the environment are generally more important because they represent a greater contributor to dose. A key feature of environmental monitoring programs for such facilities is therefore the identification of the potentially critical radionuclides that might be released, their pathways through the environment, and the avenues and mechanisms through which they might cause population exposures. Figure 11.1 shows the major steps in such a program.

Background Data

Before monitoring begins, background information is needed on other nuclear facilities in the area, the distribution and activities of the potentially exposed population, local land and water use patterns, and the local meteorology and hydrology. These data permit identification of potentially vulnerable groups, important radionuclides, and likely environmental pathways whose media can be sampled.

The background analysis must also take into account the type of installation, the nature and quantities of radioactive materials being used, their potential for release, the likely physical and chemical forms of the releases, other sources of the same contaminants in the area, and the nature of the receiving environment. This last item includes natural features (such as climate, topography, geology, and hydrology), artificial features (such as reservoirs, harbors, dams, and lakes), land use (residential, industrial, recreational, dairying, and farming of leaf or root crops), and the sources of local water supplies (surface versus groundwater). Results from a monitoring program conducted before a facility begins operation can be used to confirm these analyses and to establish baseline information for subsequent interpretation.

Radioactive materials released from a nuclear facility may end up in many sections of the environment, and their quantity and composition will vary with time and facility operation. As a result, there may

Table 11.2   Advantages and disadvantages of various environmental
sampling methods

Type of sample	Advantages	Disadvantages
Atmospheric environment		
Direct measurement		
Real-time field measurements of physical stresses such as noise and radiation	Monitors can be put in place to assess time-integrated exposures	Monitor often disturbs field being monitored; some monitoring equipment (for example, for assessing electric and magnetic fields) expensive and complex
Airborne particulates		
Respirable fraction via air sampling	Direct-dose vector; provides data on potential effects on lungs	Omits larger particles that may be significant when deposited in nose, mouth, and throat
Total particulates via air sampling	Provides data for assessing doses to lungs as well as possible effects on skin and intake through ingestion	Not all measured contaminants respirable
Collection of settled particulates	Represents an integrated sample over known time period and geographic area	Weathering may alter results; only large particles collected by sedimentation
Gases		
Integrated (concentrated) sample	Concentration of samples permits detection of lower concentrations in air	Samples must usually be analyzed in laboratory; chemical reactions may change nature of collected compounds
Direct measurement	Provides data on real-time basis	Lower limit of detection may not be adequate

Table 11.2   (continued)

Type of sample	Advantages	Disadvantages
	Terrestrial environment	
Milk	Direct-dose vector, especially for children; data easily interpreted	Milk samples not always available
Foodstuffs	Direct-dose vector; data easily interpreted	Samples not always available from areas of interest; weathering and processing may affect samples
Wildlife	Direct-dose vector	High mobility; not always available; data difficult to interpret
Vegetation	Samples readily available; multiple modes for accumulating contaminants (by direct deposition and leaf and root uptake)	Data difficult to interpret; weathering can cause loss of contaminants; not available in all seasons
Soil sampling	Good integrator of deposition over time	High analytical cost; data difficult to interpret in terms of population exposure and dose

be many pathways through which the released radionuclides can reach the public. Figures 11.2 and 11.3 outline the primary pathways, air and water. Clearly, tracing the movement of all radionuclides through all potential pathways would be physically and economically impossible. Fortunately, experience has shown that in most situations the primary contributors to population dose consist of no more than half a dozen radionuclides moving through no more than three or four pathways. Once these are identified along with the habits of the people

Table 11.2 (continued)

Type of sample	Advantages	Disadvantages
	Aquatic environment	
Surface water (non-drinking)	Readily available; indicates possibility of contamination by aquatic plants and animals	Not directly dose related; difficult to interpret data
Groundwater (non-drinking)	Indicator of unsatisfactory waste-management practices	Not always available; data difficult to interpret because of possibility of multiple remote sources
Drinking water	Direct-dose vector; consumed by all population groups	Contaminant concentrations frequently very low
Aquatic plants	Sensitivity	Data difficult to interpret; not available in all seasons
Sediment	Sensitivity; good integrator of past contamination	Data difficult to interpret because of possibility of multiple remote sources
Fish and shellfish	Direct-dose vector; sensitive indicator of contamination	Frequently unavailable; high mobility
Waterfowl	Direct-dose vector	Frequently unavailable; high mobility; data difficult to interpret

living or working in the vicinity, it should be possible to identify a "maximally exposed" group of individuals (the "critical group") whose activities and location would make them likely to receive the largest exposures. Since most countries' regulatory requirements apply to the dose to the critical group, environmental monitoring programs must be designed to provide this type of estimate. In addition, such programs must provide a means of estimating the total (collective) population dose (expressed in person-sieverts, and calculated

Table 11.3 Sources of information on environmental monitoring programs
for nuclear facilities

Agency	Document	Content
DOE	J. P. Corley et al., *A Guide for Environmental Radiological Surveillance at U.S. Department of Energy Installations*, Report DOE/EP-0023 (Springfield, Va., 1981)	Guidance on programs for DOE laboratories and contractors
EPA	*Environmental Radioactivity Surveillance Guide*, Report ORP/SID 72-2 (Washington, D.C., 1972)	One of the earliest guides: now a classic
IAEA	*Radiological Impact of Radionuclides Dispersed on a Regional and Global Scale: Methods for Assessment and Their Application*, Technical Reports Series no. 250 (Vienna, 1985)	Guidance on regional and global effects
ICRP	*Principles of Monitoring for the Radiation Protection of the Population*, Annals of the ICRP Publication 43, (New York, 1985)	Definitive information on program design
	Radionuclide Release into the Environment: Assessment of Doses to Man, Annals of the ICRP Publication 29, (New York, 1979)	General principles for dose assessments
NCRP	*Radiological Assessment: Predicting the Transport, Bioaccumulation, and Uptake by Man of Radionuclides Released to the Environment*, Report no. 76 (Bethesda, Md., 1984)	Detailed information on the environmental behavior of radionuclides
	Screening Techniques for Determining Compliance with Environmental Standards, Commentary no. 3, rev. 1 (Bethesda, Md., 1989)	Simple techniques for determining compliance
NRC	*Environmental Monitoring of Low-Level Radioactive Waste Disposal Facility*, Report NUREG-1388 (Washington, D.C., 1989)	Guidance for radioactive waste disposal facilities
	Radiological Assessment: A Textbook on Environmental Dose Analysis, Report NUREG/CR-3332 (Washington, D.C., 1983)	Detailed guidance on all aspects of environmental monitoring

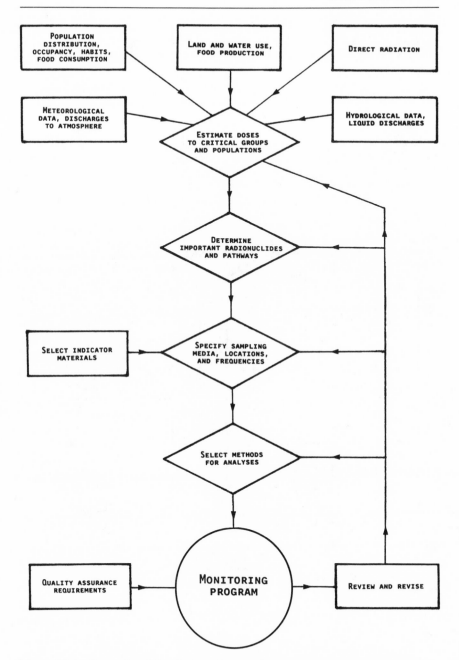

Figure 11.1 Example of the design of an environmental monitoring program and associated dose estimations for a major nuclear facility

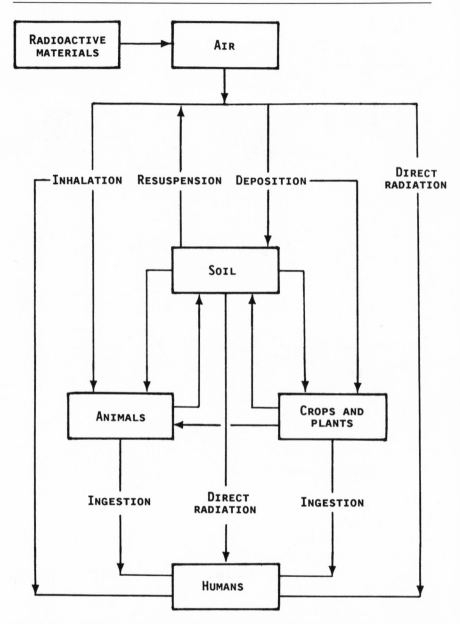

Figure 11.2   Pathways to humans for radioactive materials released into the atmosphere

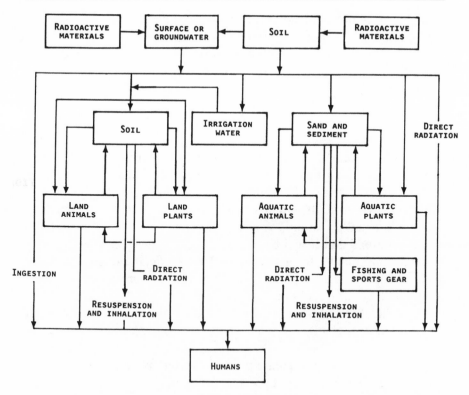

Figure 11.3 Pathways to humans for radioactive materials released to ground
or surface waters (including oceans)

by multiplying the total number of people exposed by their average
individual dose). On the basis of this estimate, regulatory authorities
can project the associated health impacts on the population as a whole
(Chapter 10).

The design principles outlined above can be applied to many environmental exposure situations. For example, a secondary lead smelter
has the potential for releasing elemental lead and associated compounds into the atmosphere, whereupon they may become an inhalation hazard. The same facility can also release these contaminants
to the soil, either directly or through the air, whereupon they may
contaminate groundwater and subsequently be taken up by fish and
agricultural products. The milk from cows and the beef from cattle
grazing on pastures adjacent to lead smelters can be expected to have

a higher-than-normal lead content. Children playing on contaminated earth near such smelters have shown elevated lead concentrations in their blood. Arsenic emitted by copper smelters follows identical pathways of contamination and human exposure.

Sample Collection and Analysis

The samples collected at a nuclear facility itself will usually contain the largest number of radionuclides at the highest concentrations (Moeller et al., 1978). However, unlike toxic chemical releases, the radioactive material will include some radionuclides that decay (and disappear) very rapidly. In contrast, samples collected in the environment will usually contain fewer radionuclides, and often in such low concentrations that it will be difficult to distinguish those released by the nuclear facility from the natural or artificial radioactive background. Analysis of in-plant samples must therefore focus on identifying and quantifying the complex mixtures likely to be present, whereas analysis of samples from the environment should be based on measurements of extremely small concentrations of preselected critical radionuclides.

In a routine environmental monitoring program, a number of trade-offs must be made to obtain adequate coverage of critical radionuclide-pathway combinations at satisfactory analytical sensitivities and costs. Under all conditions, however, it is better to collect and carefully analyze a small number of well-chosen samples, taken at key locations and providing a reliable index of environmental conditions, than to process larger numbers of poorly selected, nonrepresentative samples.

Table 11.4 ranks the relative importance of various effluent pathways for a range of typical radionuclides released from nuclear facilities according to their estimated contributions to population exposure. A difference between 1 and 2 and between 2 and 3 indicates at least an order-of-magnitude decrease in dose or sensitivity. The relative importance of a particular radionuclide-pathway combination is based on three factors: (1) its potential contribution to the dose to the critical group; (2) its potential contribution to the dose to the population outside the critical group; and (3) the ease with which the radionuclide-pathway combination can be sampled and analyzed. The pathway or sampling medium shown first in each column is considered to be the

Table 11.4 Relative importance of effluent pathways and radionuclides in contributing to population exposure

Relative importance	Radionuclide				
	Tritium	Iodine-131	Mixed fission and activation products	TRU[a]	Noble gases[b]
			Air pathway		
1	Air Milk Vegetable crops	Milk Vegetable crops	Air Vegetable crops	Air	Direct radiation Air
2	Honey Vegetation Precipitation	Air Animal thyroids Forage	Milk Direct radiation Deposition	Deposition Terrestrial biota	
3				Forage	
			Water pathway		
1	Drinking water Surface water	Drinking water Milk	Fish and shellfish	Sediment Fish and shellfish	
2	Vegetable crops Honey Groundwater	Surface water Vegetable crops Forage	Waterfowl Surface water Milk	Surface water Vegetation	
3			Sediment/soil Groundwater Terrestrial biota Forage		

a. Transuranic radionuclides, primarily plutonium-239.
b. Noble gases include radionuclides such as krypton-85, xenon-133, and radon-222.

most important (Corley et al., 1981). However, even a relative importance of 1 does not indicate that the given radionuclide-pathway combination will inevitably contribute a significant dose, nor that the particular combination will be the most important in every circumstance. Final selections of the radionuclide-pathway combinations to be emphasized in a given program must be based on operating experience and monitoring data.

Upon ingestion or inhalation, different radionuclides preferentially deposit in different body organs. As a result, estimates of the dose to the public require identification and measurement of concentrations of individual radionuclides. Besides collecting data to provide estimates of exposures to the public, a monitoring program may have to measure certain other radionuclides because of the history of operations at the site or because of specific concerns of the local population. Such measurements may be necessary regardless of the levels of exposures involved. Examples include sampling and analysis for radioactive iodine in milk near commercial nuclear power plants, for plutonium in soil near most DOE installations, for tritium in the estuary near the Savannah River Plant, and for fission products in groundwater near the Pacific Northwest Laboratories.

Careful analyses of specific radionuclides in various environmental media can also be used to determine the source of the contamination. A classic example is the use of the ratio of cesium-134 (Cs-134) to cesium-137 (Cs-137) in a sample to determine whether the contamination has resulted from discharges from a nuclear power plant or from the detonation of a nuclear device. The energy source in both cases is nuclear fission, one of the products of which is radioactive Cs-137. Also produced during the fissioning process is Cs-133, a stable isotope of cesium. If the fissioning event occurs as a result of the explosion of a nuclear device, most of the Cs-133 remains in that form. If the fissioning event occurs in a nuclear reactor, the Cs-133 remains in the reactor core for some time, it is subjected to intense neutron bombardment from subsequent fissioning events, and a portion of the Cs-133 is converted into radioactive Cs-134. Therefore, when analyses show that the radioactive cesium contamination in an environmental sample contains only very small quantities of Cs-134, one can conclude that the source of contamination was probably the detonation of a nuclear device (or a severe industrial accident), rather than releases from a nuclear power plant. Likewise, analyses for vanadium, a characteristic component of fuel oils, have been used to determine whether airborne contaminants in the environment come from the combustion of oils or coal.

Making accurate measurements of external radiation exposures from releases from a nuclear facility is particularly difficult because of the relatively high contribution from natural background radiation. Similarly, it is often difficult to measure the concentrations of artificial radionuclides in certain environmental media because of the relatively high concentrations of naturally occurring radionuclides. Under current NRC regulations, the external dose rate limit for the maximally exposed individual near a nuclear power plant is about 0.05 mSv per year. Yet the average external dose rate from naturally occurring cosmic and terrestrial radiation sources in the United States is 0.6–0.7 mSv per year. Similarly, the concentration limits in milk for key artificially produced radionuclides range from less than 0.5 to more than 5 becquerel (Bq) (from a few tens to a few hundreds of picocuries [pCi]) per liter; normal concentrations of such radionuclides are well below these values. Yet the concentration of naturally occurring radioactive potassium in milk exceeds 40 Bq (1,000 pCi) per liter.

Because they are faster and less expensive than specific radionuclide analyses for showing changes in environmental concentrations, gross measurements of radioactive materials in water and in air (in which the specific contaminating radionuclides are not identified) can be very useful as trend indicators. This is similar to the measurement of "total suspended particulates" as a surrogate for, or indicator of, the health effects of particulate substances emitted into the atmosphere. For media such as milk and food products, in which concentrations of naturally occurring radionuclides may be relatively high, gross measurements are of less value and are not recommended as part of a routine monitoring program. No attempt should be made to compare gross measurements from site to site except to identify general trends. If the radionuclide composition of the releases from a specific facility is relatively stable, gross activity may be related in a simple manner to specific radionuclide concentrations of interest, and the gross activity measurements can then be related to estimates of population dose. Such use, however, should be based on repetitive verification to assure that conditions have not changed.

Radionuclide concentrations and exposure rates observed before and after a facility is placed in operation are, in reality, distributions (rather than point values) that may and often do overlap. A measurement based on the analysis of a single sample represents one point in a distribution of similar points and has a large uncertainty associated with the most probable value. In a similar manner, defining small impacts from a nuclear facility frequently becomes a question of determining whether there is a statistical difference between the measurement of natural background, alone, and the measurement of natural background plus the contribution from the facility.

Reductions in environmental radiation required by recent standards and regulations (NRC, 1991) have increased the need for highly accurate measurements. Greater accuracy (and thus improved exposure and dose estimates) can always be achieved through collecting larger samples or using longer counting times (to provide the required statistical sensitivity). Such strategies, however, are usually costly. Although few people would disagree that measurements should be able to detect concentrations below the applicable limits, there is no general agreement as to what level of radiation exposure to people is sufficiently small to be considered negligible.

Deployment of air and water samplers and dosimeters around a site can be well worth the cost of years of maintenance and operation should an accidental release occur. This is one of the reasons the EPA requires chemical plants and oil refineries to have well-designed emergency monitoring and response plans. Where the capability for measuring chemical and radioactive contaminants exists in the same site environment, the two programs should be coordinated to provide greater efficiency and lower overall monitoring program costs. Since the behavior of certain radionuclides closely follows or is influenced by the behavior of chemically related stable elements, the use of common measurement or sampling locations, if nothing else, may permit the measurement of one constituent to serve as a tracer for or indicator of the behavior of another. Examples are the behavior of strontium-90 relative to stable calcium and the behavior of cesium-137 relative to potassium.

Temporal Relationships

For each type of release from a nuclear facility, there is a characteristic pattern between the time of the release and the occurrence of

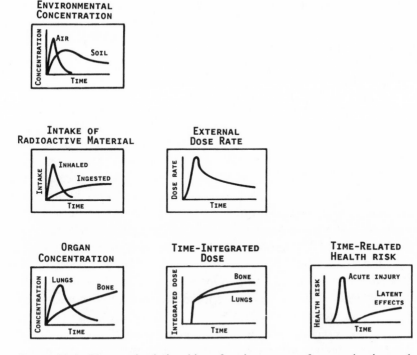

Figure 11.4   Temporal relationships of various types of contamination and accompanying human exposures resulting from environmental releases of radioactive materials

exposures (Figure 11.4). People exposed to an airborne release will immediately receive external exposures from the radionuclides within the cloud and will almost immediately inhale radioactive material and expose the lungs. Deposition of radioactive material from the cloud onto the soil will take longer, and uptake by agricultural crops and pasture grass longer still. Exposures to the bone and other organs such as the thyroid will be delayed, pending uptake and transfer of the material from the lungs. Likewise, exposures to specific organs, other than the stomach and gastrointestinal tract resulting from the ingestion of radioactive material in milk or food, will be delayed until the material is taken up by the blood and deposited in specific body organs. Acute effects from environmental exposures will appear within hours to weeks (depending on the dose); delayed effects (such as latent cancers) from lower-level exposures will not appear until some years later.

Quality Assurance Requirements

To be effective, an environmental monitoring program must be supported by a sound quality assurance program. Such a program must include (1) acceptance testing or qualification of laboratory and field sampling and analytic devices; (2) routine calibrations of all associated instrumentation, including flow measurements on field sampling equipment; (3) a laboratory cross-check program; (4) replicate sampling on a systematic basis; (5) procedural audits; and (6) documentation of laboratory and field procedures and quality-assurance records.

Sampling validity and sample preservation also need to be addressed as part of the quality assurance program. Useful tools for maintaining analytic validity include duplicate sample analyses and control charts. As a general rule, approximately 10–15 percent of the samples processed in a laboratory should be resubmitted for analysis as "blind" duplicates. Standard solutions (large bulk samples that have been analyzed so frequently that their chemical content is well established) should routinely be used to check the accuracy of new data.

Through services provided by the EPA, the National Institute for Occupational Safety and Health, and the National Institute for Standards and Technology, laboratories conducting environmental radionuclide analyses can obtain standard and cross-check samples, as well as guidance in establishing and operating a quality assurance program. The NRC requires all laboratories performing analyses of environmental samples from commercial nuclear power plants to participate in the EPA program or its equivalent. Whenever discrepancies are noted, follow-up action is required to determine and eliminate the causes.

Estimating the Dose to the Population

Experience has shown that human exposures to pollutants can differ significantly from what might be predicted solely on the basis of measurements of their concentrations in media such as air, water, soil, and food. For this reason, the design of many environmental monitoring programs has been modified in recent years to concentrate on the need to measure total human exposures. To do this, two complementary conceptual models are being used (Ott, 1990).

Direct Approach

This approach is applicable when the objective is to determine the exposures to a large population group whose individual members live within a common geographic area, have relatively similar living habits, and are thought to be exposed to similar environmental stresses. Through appropriate statistical sampling techniques, a representative sample of the target population is identified. Through the use of 24-hour personal monitors that can be worn continuously or placed next to the person being monitored, data are then obtained on airborne exposures to individual members of the same population. These data are combined with information on the concentrations of specific contaminants in food and water and with detailed data on their intake to estimate exposures to the sample population group and, in turn, exposures to the total population group.

Indirect Approach

In many situations it is desirable to use monitoring data, collected under one set of circumstances, to estimate exposures to population groups whose living habits and exposure sources are known to be different. This is much more complicated than the direct approach, and its successful application requires additional types of information. This includes data not only on the variety of schedules and activities of the people whose exposures are to be estimated, but also on the likely concentrations of various airborne pollutants in areas where they spend most of their time, such as at home, in school, in an occupational or recreational setting, or while commuting. As with the direct approach, these data must be supplemented by information on other possible avenues of exposure, including the concentrations of specific contaminants in food and water. Once this is done, models must be developed and validated for using these data to estimate the exposures to the larger population group.

Many guides exist for calculating the doses to the public from exposures to radiation and radioactive materials in the environment. The NRC's Regulatory Guide 1.109 (1977) provides a detailed methodology for making such calculations. The EPA has developed similar guidance for calculating doses from acutely toxic chemicals and carcinogens. All such calculations are generally derived using computer models that incorporate information on the key parameters described above. The choice of model is usually based on the computer available, the type and complexity of radionuclide releases, the environmental pathways associated with the specific site or facility, and the living habits of the people being exposed. Because of the different assumptions and modeling approaches used in developing the programs, different codes will frequently yield different estimates of the associated doses. Reviews of the major calculational models being used for dose assessments of environmental releases show that initial efforts in such assessments were directed primarily to atmospheric dispersion, external dosimetry, and internal dosimetry resulting from inhalation. The more recent incorporation of terrestrial and aquatic food-chain pathways reflects the desire to assess total exposure and the need to satisfy more stringent regulatory requirements.

Dose estimates made using computer models serve as a basis not only for epidemiological studies and tort litigation but also for demonstrating compliance with environmental radionuclide emission standards and guides. With the expanded use of microcomputers such models are finding widespread application in designing defensible and efficient monitoring programs and in performing associated engineering calculations. Accompanying this development is an emphasis on models that are less complex and easier to use (Till, 1988). Many of the screening models developed by the NCRP (1989) for radionuclide assessment are being modified for use in the assessment of nonradioactive environmental pollutants.

The many environmental monitoring programs under way are generating a wealth of data. The NRC annually publishes summaries of radionuclide releases and estimates of the associated population doses from the operation of commercial nuclear power plants in the United States. Estimates of population doses from government-operated nuclear facilities are published by the DOE, and the EPA reports on the concentrations of various pollutants, including toxic chemicals, in the ambient environment (EPA, 1989).

The General Outlook

Advances in computer technology and in analytic techniques promise continued improvements in environmental monitoring capabilities.

With the recognition that people spend most of their time indoors, there will be increasing emphasis on indoor monitoring, particularly of airborne pollutants. Since some of these arise from outdoor sources, there will also continue to be a need for measurements in the ambient environment. Such measurements will also be necessary to assess the concentrations of key contaminants in water and food and to assess the potential long-term effects of contaminants such as carbon dioxide (relative to the greenhouse effect), chlorofluorocarbons (relative to the destruction of the protective ozone layer), and sulfur oxides (relative to acidic deposition).

With continuous improvements in small, economical, lightweight, personal monitors, there will also undoubtedly be increased reliance on such devices for assessing human exposures. At the same time, advances in remote sensing and monitoring instruments may make it possible to determine more accurately and more simply the condition of many elements in the environment. As these better data bases are established, they will require better integration and more systematic methods of compilation and storage for use in studies of the long-term health effects of various environmental contaminants. Computer models will need to be refined not only to predict human exposures but also to assess the long-range effects of key environmental contaminants and to calculate the interrelationships among environmental factors.

Experimentation with new monitoring approaches should continue. Examples include the use of bacteria to detect organic contaminants, the use of pigeons as sensors of lead pollution, the analysis of honey as a possible indicator of releases of arsenic, cadmium, and fluoride (since bees cover large areas and collect pollen from a wide range of plants) (Bromenshenk et al., 1985), and the analysis of human hair from barbershops to screen for exposures to lead and radioactive strontium.

Environmental monitoring programs conducted by state and local regulatory and public health agencies are essential to provide an independent check on the consistency of compliance by industrial and federal governmental facilities. Such surveillance should be supplemented by periodic reevaluations in response to quantitative and qualitative modifications in effluent releases, new developments in analytic techniques and equipment, improved knowledge of the behavior of specific contaminants within the environment, new patterns of environmental use and population distribution, and changes in regulatory requirements. Periodic reviews are also necessary to address the cost effectiveness of certain kinds of sampling, so that those that do not measure relevant pathways or contain less-than-measurable quantities can be discontinued. When new measurement techniques or sampling locations are incorporated in a new program, however, sufficient overlapping data must be obtained, using the earlier techniques and locations, to provide continuity.

Recognizing the value of a strong independent environmental monitoring capability on the part of the states, the U.S. Department of Energy (DOE) initiated a program in May 1991 to provide financial support for state monitoring programs. These funds have enabled states in which major DOE facilities are located to develop and maintain well-staffed, up-to-date programs.

References

Bromenshenk, J. J., S. R. Carlson, J. C. Simpson, and J. M. Thomas. 1985. "Pollution Monitoring of Puget Sound with Honey Bees." *Science* 227 (8 February), 632–634.

Corley, J. P., D. H. Denham, R. E. Jaquish, D. E. Michels, A. R. Olsen, and D. A. Waite. 1981. *A Guide for Environmental Radiological Surveillance at U.S. Department of Energy Installations*. Report DOE/EP-0023. Springfield, Va.: U.S. Department of Energy, National Technical Information Service.

EPA. 1989. *The Toxics-Release Inventory: A National Perspective*. Report EPA 560/4-89-005. Washington, D.C.

Moeller, D. W., J. M. Selby, D. A. Waite, and J. P. Corley. 1978. "Environmental Surveillance for Nuclear Facilities." *Nuclear Safety* 19, no. 1 (January–February), 66–79.

NCRP. 1989. *Screening Techniques for Determining Compliance with Environmental Standards*. Commentary no. 3, Revision 1. Bethesda, Md.

NRC. 1977. *Calculation of Annual Doses to Man from Routine Releases of Reactor Effluents for the Purpose of Evaluating Compliance with 10 CFR Part 50, Appendix I*. Regulatory Guide 1.109. Washington, D.C.

——— 1991. "Standards for Protection against Radiation." Code of Federal Regulations, Title 10, Part 20.

Ott, Wayne R. 1990. "Total Human Exposure: Basic Concepts, EPA Field Studies, and Future Research Needs." *Journal of the Air & Waste Management Association* 40, no. 7 (July), 966–975.

Till, J. E. 1988. "Modeling the Outdoor Environment—New Perspectives and Challenges." *Health Physics* 55, no. 2 (August), 331–338.

12

Energy

Meeting energy needs and protecting the environment are inseparable. If energy needs are to be met, care must be taken to assure that the public health and safety, as well as the environment, are protected. The mining of coal, for example, can lead to chronic diseases and injuries among miners and to degradation of the environment (as is often the case in strip mining); the drilling, acquisition, and transportation of oil can lead to spills that contaminate vast areas of land, water, or both; and the combustion of gasoline in cars leads to air pollution and smog. Internationally, the production and use of oil can lead to conflicts among nations and even to wars. The generation of electricity through either hydropower or the combustion of fossil or nuclear fuels leads to air pollution, problems of waste disposal, and other effects on the environment. Added to these concerns is the need to consider the long-range impacts, such as acidic deposition and the greenhouse effect (ASME, 1989), of the burning of fossil fuels (Chapter 14).

Conservation can play a major role in meeting energy needs. One of the most obvious places to practice conservation is the home, currently the source of one-sixth of the energy consumed in the United States. Newer generations of technology are leading to far more efficient ways to light, cool, and heat dwellings. Other improvements include the installation of more efficient appliances. These conservation measures have been made a part of construction techniques for new buildings. Such actions, however, are not always without negative impacts; examples are increased radon concentrations and the "sick building syndrome" (ASME, 1989). Even the use of solar energy has associated problems. These range from occupational health problems in the manufacture of photovoltaic cells, to injuries and deaths to home owners who fall while cleaning solar panels on the roofs of their houses.

An adequate supply of energy is important to the health and comfort of people throughout the world. Yet before 1973 few Americans were aware that the supplies of some fuels are limited. This fact was forced on their attention then by an oil embargo, and accompanying increases in gasoline prices, and again in 1990 and early 1991 by the Persian Gulf conflict. Before 1973 most people in the United States thought they could live indefinitely in what some have called a "logarithmic" world; that is, one in which they could have an expanding economy accompanied by a continuing increase in the world's population and the use of energy, with concurrent increases in the consumption of food and material goods.

Now most policymakers recognize that the world's energy and environmental resources are limited and that continued health and safety will be possible only if these resources are carefully managed, conserved, and protected. Since higher standards of living invariably require increased uses of energy, people in the developing nations can move forward only if they have access to a fair share of the world's limited energy resources. Today the United States, with only about 6 percent of the world's population, consumes about 30 percent of the world's energy. It imports more oil than France, Germany, Italy, the Netherlands, and the United Kingdom combined, and three times as much oil as Japan. For the foreseeable future, 50 percent of the oil consumed in the United States will be imported. Of this amount, 40 percent is used for transportation. And since there is currently no readily available substitute for gasoline or oil for American cars, trucks, airplanes, and diesel locomotives, our entire transportation system is vulnerable to the continued availability of these imported supplies. Fortunately, the Clean Air Act of 1990 requires that alternate fuels be developed for use in automobiles and trucks. Although this requirement is based on reductions in engine emissions, it should also reduce our dependence on foreign oil.

Energy Uses in the United States

Making long-range plans for meeting energy needs requires detailed knowledge of current energy sources and how they are being used. Today, 23 percent of the energy consumed in the United States is used by industry, 29 percent for transportation, 11 percent for commercial or residential purposes, and 37 percent by electric utilities (Council on Environmental Quality, 1989).

Industrial

About half of the energy used in industry is for heating processes, either through direct burning of fuels or through the generation of steam. Much of the remainder is used for operating machinery, lighting, and manufacturing processes. About three-quarters of all energy used in manufacturing is consumed by six highly consumptive industrial groups: chemicals (including the manufacture of plastics) use 30 percent; petroleum refining, 28 percent; the production of metals such as aluminum and steel, 21 percent; the manufacture of paper, stone, glass, and clay products, 16 percent; and food processing, 5 percent.

Transportation

There are about 120 million automobiles in the United States, approximately one for every two members of the population. Although federal regulations have required the production of more-energy-efficient cars, the government has also subsidized the construction of thousands of miles of highways that have encouraged people to drive more and to consume more fuel. Exacerbating this trend is a general lack of support for the development of mass transportation systems. Automobiles currently account for 95 percent of all urban commuting, although trains and buses can transport people at half or less the energy consumption per person-mile.

With the deregulation of airlines, airplanes have become the fastest-growing mode of intercity passenger transport, although they consume far more energy per person-mile than a car and vastly more than a bus or train. Freight transportation has followed a similar trend. Rail transport is 4 times as efficient as truck transport and more than 60 times as efficient as air transport, but railroads are continuing to lose freight traffic to trucks and airplanes.

Although American-made cars now average more than twice as many miles per gallon as in the mid-1970s, other factors have kept overall gains below what they might have been. Additional controls on engine emissions have exacted a penalty on fuel economy. There is increased use of energy-consuming features such as air conditioning and power steering. Although the use of lighter-weight metals and materials, such as aluminum and plastics, has led to better fuel economy, the manufacture of these materials requires more energy than the manufacture of traditional metals (General Motors, 1990). These changes will also affect the environmental impact of the car's ultimate disposal (Chapter 6).

Residential

Reflecting a trend toward smaller housing units and the desire of both older and younger people to live in homes of their own, the number of households in the United States has been increasing more rapidly than the population. As a result, residential energy use has increased dramatically. A typical house contains five basic energy-consuming items: a central heating system, a hot-water heater, a stove for cooking, a refrigerator, and a lighting system. In addition many contain air-conditioners, dish washers, clothes washers and dryers, television sets, tape recorders, personal computers, or some combination of these. Accompanying an increase in the number of these appliances is an increase in the consumption of energy. For example, dish and clothes washers consume electricity not only directly but also indirectly, in their demand on hot water; frost-free refrigerators use 60 percent more electricity than earlier models; color television sets require about 50 percent more electricity than black-and-white sets; and electric stoves, though less polluting, require about three times as much energy as natural gas stoves (since electricity-generating plants operate at about 35 percent efficiency).

Somewhat offsetting this trend has been the increased use of microwave ovens, which require only about one-third to one-half as much energy as conventional ovens. Similarly, today's personal computers are smaller and consume far less energy than earlier models.

Commercial

Commercial uses of energy include such diverse operations as stores, office buildings, hotels, gasoline stations, schools, hospitals, theaters, restaurants, and sports arenas. For the past several decades, increases in this sector have been greater than those in industry.

Most of the energy consumption in commercial buildings is for space heating and cooling, lighting, and office equipment. Because of the trend to sealed windows (which require continuous ventilation), higher lighting levels, glass curtain walls (which permit significant heat loss and gain), and the proliferation of computers, elevators, escalators, and duplicating machines, office buildings constructed in recent years tend to use far more energy than older buildings. The World Trade Center in New York City, comprising two buildings and housing a working population of 50,000, consumes as much electricity as Syracuse, New York, with a population of 175,000 (Gore, 1981).

Energy Resources

The fuels available to meet the world's energy needs include renewable sources, such as solar energy (including wind and waterpower) and geothermal energy, and nonrenewable sources, such as fossil fuels (coal, oil, and natural gas) and nuclear fuels (such as uranium and plutonium) (ASME, 1989). Fusion reactors, like solar energy, could represent an almost limitless source.

Fossil Fuels

Experience shows that when fossil fuels are first discovered, they are used at a very modest level. Their use then increases more or less continuously to a maximum and thereafter declines to zero when available supplies have been consumed (Hubbert, 1973). Both in the United States and worldwide, production (consumption) of oil and natural gas has probably already peaked and is now on a downward curve. Production and consumption of coal are still on the increase. The remaining supplies of these three fuels are estimated to be about as follows:

Natural gas: perhaps one to two decades; however, new supplies are being discovered, and the total recoverable reserves are probably not known at this time.

Oil (petroleum): perhaps three to five decades; more than half of these resources are located in the Middle East.

Coal: perhaps two to four centuries; the United States has abundant reserves.

Nuclear Fuel

The energy available through existing sources of uranium, if consumed exclusively in the current generation of boiling and pressurized water nuclear power plants, is estimated to be about equal to that available through the combustion of existing sources of natural gas or petroleum. With the development of breeder reactors (and the recycling of plutonium), nuclear fuel could become a far larger energy source than any of the fossil fuels (Figure 12.1). Even so, none of these sources begins to approach the amount of energy that would be made available by effective harnessing of the fusion process. In contrast to the fission process, which involves splitting the nuclei of heavy elements and is the basic process involved in the operation of nuclear power plants, fusion involves the combination of very small (or light) nuclei. Both processes result in significant releases of energy. The fusion process, for example, is the source of energy in the sun and the stars. Control of the fusion process would make water the main source of energy through the combination of the deuterium, or heavy hydrogen atoms, it contains to form helium. This process can take place only at extremely high temperatures and has not yet been achieved on a controlled basis.

Solar Energy

Solar sources offer tremendous potential for meeting the world's energy needs. Since solar energy is renewable, once a given use is established it can be applied more or less indefinitely.

Sources of solar energy include wind and waterpower, use of sunlight as a heat source, conversion of agricultural crops into fuels, and direct conversion into electricity.

One of the most common applications of solar energy is the use of hydropower to generate electricity (such as the enormously successful series of hydroelectric power plants constructed in the mid-twentieth century by the Tennessee Valley Authority). However, experience with the Aswan High Dam in Egypt (discussed below) has shown that hydroelectric plants can have major impacts on environmental and public health. In the United States, there are few acceptable sites left for large hydropower plants, so the potential for further development of this source is limited to small-scale hydroelectric projects.

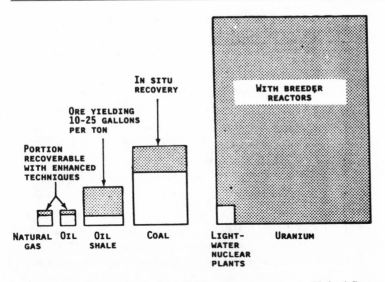

Figure 12.1 Comparison of available energy resources, United States

Another possible application of waterpower is the harnessing of the tides. Although a proposal in the early 1960s to construct such a plant in the Bay of Fundy, in Maine, was not approved, other countries are using this resource, an example being the tidal electric power station now being built in the United Kingdom.

Another possibility is to harness the wind with arrays of windmills located in a common area. Although windmills have been used for centuries on an individual basis to pump water, few multiunit wind-power stations have been developed so far. This situation, however, may be changing. California now has three wind-power turbine plants, and studies by the Electric Power Research Institute (Schaefer, 1989) indicate that wind power may offer electric utilities a pollution-free system that is cost-competitive with conventional sources. Some experts estimate that there are enough windy areas in the United States to meet as much as 25 percent of the country's electricity needs (Shea, 1988). Plans for large-scale wind farms are now under way in Germany and the United Kingdom (Dickson, 1989; Kirk, 1989).

Similar progress has been reported in the construction and installation of large collectors for the direct conversion of sunlight into electricity (EPRI, 1989). The use of solar collectors to provide power for small appliances, such as sun-powered watches, typewriters, calculators, and answering machines, has also been very successful and is seeing widespread application. Patio walkway lights that store the sun's energy during the day and release it at night have also proved popular. In addition, solar-powered units are being widely used to serve remote installations such as offshore oil-drilling equipment, microwave transformers, navigational lights, and signal buoys (Somerville, 1989). It will probably be some time, however, before major units can be developed for widescale conversion of sunlight into electricity. Cost and land use remain major obstacles (ASME, 1989).

In some parts of the world fuel is being produced from various agricultural crops. For example, ethanol can be made from sugar cane, methanol can be made from wood materials, methane can be produced by the anaerobic disgestion of animal and plant wastes, and biomass (particularly wood and wood waste) can be directly burned as a fuel.

The potential applications of solar energy extend far beyond these examples. The selection of the trees that are planted around a house can promote not only comfort but also energy conservation. Deciduous trees, for example, can provide shade in the summer and permit sunlight to warm the house in the winter. In the developing countries the sun is used for heating and distilling water, for drying crops, and for heat engines such as the SOFRETES pump, manufactured in France.

Geothermal Energy

Geothermal energy is thought to be produced by the radioactive decay of naturally occurring radionuclides in the rocks beneath the earth's surface. Although the quantity of geothermal energy is enormous, it is often difficult to tap and is limited to certain geographic areas. In the United States, these areas are primarily in the West, where geothermal energy is the source of many hot-water and natural steam reservoirs. In many areas the underground reservoirs of hot water are directly tapped to provide heat for residences, businesses, and industrial processes. In Boise, Idaho, for example, the water from hot springs has been used to heat homes since the 1890s (Anonymous, 1981). Where steam is present, geothermal energy can be used to generate electricity. In fact, plants in the Geysers field in California produce as much electricity as several large nuclear power plants

(National Research Council, 1979). Where water is not present, the heat may simply be stored in dry rock, and some method (for example, pumping water through the rock) would have to be used for extracting it.

Although progress in harnessing geothermal energy sources has been slow, more than 2 million acres of federal land have been leased for exploration and development (Anonymous, 1981). Unfortunately, most of the accessible, higher-grade hot-water reservoirs are in areas remote from population and industry. As a result, the main potential of geothermal energy in the United States appears to lie in localized use as a source of inexpensive heat on a relatively small scale. Because steam can be transported only a few miles without enormous energy losses, there is little large-scale market for the heat unless it can be converted into electricity. And there are very few commercial-size steam reservoirs, such as the Geysers, that can be used to generate electricity in the United States (National Research Council, 1979). Worldwide, however, there are many opportunities for generating electricity with geothermal energy sources. Prime sites exist in Central America and parts of Southeast Asia, East Africa, and southern Europe. The Philippines and Mexico have developed electricity-generating stations at several major geothermal fields (Flavin, 1986).

Environmental Impacts

The National Environmental Policy Act of 1969 requires assessments of the potential environmental and public health impacts of all new major commercial and industrial facilities. Such assessments must include an analysis of data on the existing environment, as well as analyses of the facility's potential effects on it. Data on the existing environment can be obtained from previous records and from a monitoring program in the area in which the facility is to be located (Chapter 11). Information on potential impacts can be obtained from data on the impacts of existing comparable facilities elsewhere. The projected impacts must be in compliance with the standards or limits for various chemical substances and other contaminants in the environment (Chapter 10). The assessment must also include analyses of any unavoidable adverse effects should the facility be built, the range of available alternatives, and any irreversible and irretrievable commitments of resources.

In any discussion of energy use, one topic that inevitably arises is the environmental impact of electricity-generating power plants. In plants using coal and oil, smoke from the tall stacks is clearly visible and thus easily subject to public comment. Nuclear power, the major alternative to coal and oil, remains a highly emotional and controversial subject. Yet demand for electricity continues to grow. Of the total energy consumed in the United States, almost 40 percent is used in the form of electricity (Council on Environmental Quality, 1989). Figure 12.2 shows the relative increase in population, electricity consumption, and total energy use in the United States since 1950, with projections to the year 2000. Here, as in many other countries, the use of electricity has far outstripped population growth or total energy use: in 1973–1988 alone, the use of electricity in the United States increased by 54 percent.

The following sections assess and compare the environmental impacts of various methods of generating electricity: hydroelectric power, geothermal energy, fossil-fueled power plants, and nuclear-powered plants.

Hydroelectric Power

Harnessing waterpower on a major scale generally involves the construction of a dam on a river or stream. This forms a lake, and the potential energy in the water in the lake is used to turn turbines and to generate electricity. Many people consider hydroelectric power to have the least harmful effects on the environment. But experience has shown that large-scale projects can alter the environment, and people's lives, drastically, bringing as many risks as benefits. The Aswan High Dam on the Nile River in Egypt exemplifies the problems that can accompany the development and use of hydroelectric power. The Aswan project had two objectives in damming the Nile: to produce electric power and to irrigate the nearby desert, thereby producing vast amounts of new farmland. But there were many unforeseen results.

First, when flowing in its original state, the Nile carried a tremendous quantity of silt and organic matter all the way to its mouth each year, and this material attracted great numbers of fish. In 1964, for example, 31,000 tons of fish were caught near the mouth of the river. In 1968, after construction of the dam was completed, less food mate-

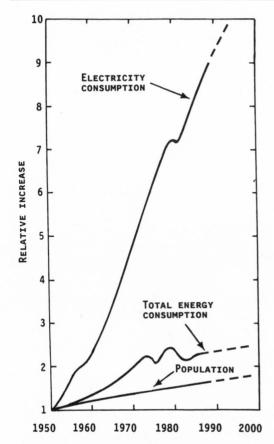

Figure 12.2 Relative increase in U.S population, total energy use, and electricity consumption (data normalized to 1950)

rial was discharged into the Mediterranean, only 500 tons of fish were caught, and 4,500 fishermen were put out of work (White, 1988).

Second, in its original state the Nile flooded the plains along its banks every spring. The deposition of silt and organic matter (an estimated 500 million tons per year) in these areas made them excellent farmlands. Once the dam was built, the river no longer flooded the plains, no silt and organic matter were deposited, and the fertility of these areas declined. In addition, the dam raised the water table under the land around the lake behind the dam. This water, in turn, dissolved salts in the ground and brought them up to the topsoil, making it less usable for agriculture than anticipated. The initial loss of farmland downstream was greater than the amount gained upriver through the use of irrigation from water in the lake behind the dam. Even today there is still a small net loss in agricultural acreage (White, 1988). In addition, control of the flow rate in the river led to increased growth of algae and phytoplankton, which adversely affected water quality. Quiescence also promoted the growth of snails, with a dramatic increase in the incidence of schistosomiasis among people living nearby.

Third, as a result of the flooding of the area above the dam, 50,000–100,000 people and the ancient temple at Abu Simbel had to be relocated.

Finally, the sudden failure of a dam can have catastrophic effects in terms of loss of livelihoods and lives. For example, more than 400 people were killed in the failure of the Malpasset dam, in southern France, during a flood in 1959. Recent evidence shows that, although the potential seismic impacts may not have been properly considered in the construction of the Aswan High Dam, the facility should be able to withstand the earthquakes anticipated in that area (White, 1988).

Geothermal Energy

As is the case for other energy sources, the use of geothermal energy has a variety of environmental impacts. The pressure in pressurized hot-water reservoirs is often a result of the weight of the overlying land; withdrawal of the water can lead to subsidence. This concern limits exploitation of many such reservoirs. Accidental spills of the withdrawn water, which often has a high mineral content, can lead to soil salination and water pollution. Where water is injected to be converted into steam using the heat from dry rocks, there will be some risk of induced seismicity (National Research Council, 1979).

The major geothermal energy sources being tapped for the generation of electricity are steam reservoirs. In most cases the steam is quite pure and can be piped directly from a well to a turbine generator system. At the electricity-generating stations at the Geysers, however, the condensed steam must be reinjected after use because it contains harmful chemicals. Because the quantities of water involved are small, withdrawal of the steam does not lead to problems of subsidence (National Research Council, 1979). In addition to these impacts, there may be significant problems from the release of radon and volatile gases, such as hydrogen sulfide, that accompany the steam. The quantities of radon being released from such operations in northern California equal or exceed the airborne releases for other types of radionuclides from nuclear-powered plants of comparable generating capacity (Hellums, 1990).

Use of Nuclear or Fossil Fuels

Facilities that generate electric power with nuclear or fossil fuels use similar processes. In both cases the fuel is used to produce heat, which converts water to steam. The steam is then sent to a turbine, which is connected to a generator for producing electricity. Cooling water, usually from a nearby river or lake, is used to condense the steam leaving the discharge side of the turbine, and the hot water is then returned to the heat source for reheating. Condensation of the steam leaving the turbine produces a vacuum so that the incoming steam will have the necessary pressure to turn the turbines. In this process, twice as much energy—that is, twice as much heat—is discharged to the environment with the cooling water as is converted into electricity, and power plants of this type are increasingly being challenged as sources of thermal pollution. Such plants also release various gases and particles into the atmosphere, along with smaller quantities of liquid wastes.

To avoid thermal pollution of water sources, many electric utilities have equipped their power plants with cooling towers, which release the excess heat into the atmosphere instead of into a lake or river. During cold weather the steam leaving the towers can condense and freeze on nearby roads and cause accidents. Some scientists have speculated that a large number of cooling towers, concentrated in so-called power parks, could cause local changes in the weather.

Both fossil-fueled and nuclear-fueled power plants have environmental impacts at five stages:

Fuel acquisition
Fuel transportation
Power plant releases
Processing and disposal of spent fuel or ashes
Power transmission

Fuel Acquisition

Acquisition of fossil fuels has considerable environmental impacts. In the case of coal and oil these are largely related to the volumes required. For example, a standard 1,000-megawatt electric (MWe) power plant requires more than 2 million tons of coal or more than 500 million gallons of oil per year.

Strip mining of coal pollutes the air with dust and defaces the earth's surface, if the land is not restored to its original state after the mining process is completed. Underground mining of coal frequency produces "acid mine drainage"—sulfuric acid and iron salts that drain out of or seep from the mine during operation and for some years thereafter. When these materials flow into surface steams, they are toxic to most forms of aquatic life. And coal miners experience an array of occupational health problems. Ten percent or more of working coal miners today show evidence of coal miner's pneumoconiosis; twice that number show evidence of other types of respiratory illnesses. More than 420,000 federal compensation awards were made to coal miners between 1970 and the end of 1977, in the amount of about $1 billion annually (Office of Technology Assessment, 1979). The mining of a sufficient quantity of coal to provide fuel for one 1,000-MWe power station results in 2–4 accidental deaths and 2–8 cases of black lung disease and other respiratory diseases among coal miners each year (Wrenn, 1979).

Drilling for oil has environmental impacts both on land and offshore. Oil refineries release airborne wastes, and leaks from offshore drilling operations can contaminate the marine environment. Notable examples were the spills some years ago near Santa Barbara, California, and more recently in the Gulf of Mexico and the North Sea.

Underground mining of uranium can also have serious effects on health. Of the 6,000 people who have worked or are now working in uranium mines in the United States, an estimated 15–20 percent, or about 1,000, have already died or will die from lung cancer within the next 10–20 years. Most of the exposures leading to these deaths occurred in the years immediately before and after World War II, before standards were established and controls implemented. Fortunately, because the total quantity of fuel required is so small, the mining of the uranium required to fuel a 1,000-MWe nuclear power plant is estimated to cause only about 0.1 accidental death, and 0–0.4

delayed occupational death, per year (Wrenn, 1979). However, the processing of uranium ore produces large quantities of tailings that can be sources of liquid and gaseous releases to the environment (Chapter 6).

Fuel Transportation

A standard 1,000-MWe coal-fired electric power plant requires about 8,000 tons of fuel per day, enough to fill at least 100 railroad cars. The transportation of this amount of coal is estimated to result in 2–4 deaths and 25–40 injuries each year, primarily as a result of accidents at railroad crossings (Gotchy, 1987). For this and economic reasons, the concept of the "mine-mouth power plant" is being implemented for coal-fired plants in several western states. Under this approach, the power plant is constructed near the source of the coal. Although the electricity must subsequently be transmitted over greater distances, this strategy is considered preferable to transporting the coal.

Far more notorious are the environmental problems associated with the transportation of oil. Much of the oil consumed in the United States is obtained overseas, and tanker accidents are common. The wreck of the *Torrey Canyon* in 1967 spilled about 30 million gallons of oil into the English Channel and onto nearby beaches; the accident involving the *Exxon Valdez* to Prince William Sound, Alaska, in the spring of 1989 released more than 10 million gallons. Most tanker accidents occur within 10 miles of shore, they usually affect a recreational area, and the average amount of oil spilled is more than 25,000 barrels, or more than 1 million gallons per accident. The cost of cleanup is substantial; in the case of the *Exxon Valdez* spill, it exceeded $2 billion.

The ocean shipment of natural gas poses similar problems (Martino, 1980). A modern tanker can transport about 125,000 cubic meters of liquefied natural gas at a temperature of −160°C. When the tanker reaches its destination, the liquified gas is allowed to warm and regassify as it is transferred to storage tanks for later distribution to consumers. During this process the volume of the gas increases by more than 600 percent. An accident while a tanker is unloading its cargo could release millions of cubic meters of natural gas (in expanded cloud form) as a blanket over a city. If the cloud were later ignited, widespread death and destruction would result.

In theory, a 1,000-MWe plant powered by nuclear fuel requires only about one ton of fuel per year. However, since the fuel cannot be entirely consumed because it becomes contaminated with fission products, the actual amount of fuel required is closer to 30–50 tons per year. Because the original uranium fuel is sealed within fuel rods and does not represent an external radiation source, its transportation to the power plant does not represent any unusual occupational or environmental health problems.

Power Plant Releases

Fossil-fueled plants release sulfur oxides, nitrogen oxides, carbon monoxide, and some radioactive material originating naturally in the fuel (Wilson et al., 1981). In fact, the United Nations Scientific Committee on the Effects of Atomic Radiation estimates that the collective dose from a coal-fired electricity-generating plant is equivalent to 25 percent of the local and regional population dose from a nuclear-powered station of the same generating capacity (Mettler et al., 1990). Fossil-fueled plants also release significant amounts of carbon dioxide into the atmosphere. Table 12.1 summarizes the estimated quantities of major airborne pollutants released by coal-, oil-, and gas-fired 1,000-MWe plants. The numbers, which vary depending on a range of plant conditions and are presented primarily for purposes of illustration, indicate that oil-fired plants discharge more than twice as many sulfur oxides as coal-fired plants. Gas-fired plants emit essentially no sulfur oxides. Coal-fired plants release more than twice as much nitrogen oxide as oil-fired plants, and almost four times as much as plants fueled by natural gas. Coal-fired plants release two to three times as much carbon monoxide as plants fueled by oil or natural gas. And both the coal- and oil-fired plants discharge four to five times as many particulates as plants fueled with natural gas.

Clearly, a plant fueled by natural gas has far less impact on the environment than a plant fueled by coal or oil. Why, then, do public utilities not use natural gas as their sole source of fuel for generating electricity? The answer is twofold: there does not seem to be enough natural gas available to meet such a demand, and the fuel can be used more effectively for other purposes, such as home heating. Even so, many power plants have installed natural gas turbine systems to handle periods of peak demand. Although facilities for converting coal

Table 12.1 Airborne emissions from fossil-fueled electric power plants (assumed capacity 1,000 MWe)

Pollutant	Emission (tons per day)[a]		
	Coal	Oil	Natural gas
Sulfur oxides	12	32	0.06
Nitrogen oxides	86	36	23
Carbon monoxide	6	2.5	1.8
Particulates	3.6	4.6	1

a. Emissions will vary depending on nature of fuel, plant design, and operating parameters.

into gas have been considered, such conversion has not yet proved to be cost-effective on a large-scale commercial basis.

The kind and quantity of releases from nuclear-powered plants depend on the type of reactor. Two basic types are in use in the United States today: pressurized water reactors (PWRs) and boiling water reactors (BWRs) (Figure 12.3). In a BWR the water is heated by the fuel and converted into steam, and this steam turns the turbine. Neutron irradiation of the cooling water as it passes through the reactor core converts stable oxygen into radioactive nitrogen, which is then carried by the steam out to the turbine. As a result, personnel cannot work in the vicinity of the turbine during plant operation. If there are leaks in the fuel cladding, the water and steam will also contain radioactive fission products.

In a PWR the water heated by the reactor is kept under sufficient pressure that it is not converted into steam. Through use of an intermediate heat exchanger (steam generator) this water, in turn, transfers heat to water in a secondary system, which is converted into steam and turns the turbine. Under normal conditions the water in the secondary system will be clean, and any leakage will not involve the release of radioactive material. However, the tubing in the steam generators frequently fails, releasing radioactive water and gases from the primary to the secondary system. Although the liquid releases can be readily controlled, some gases are released to the environment.

Contrary to what one would expect, airborne releases from a BWR are smaller than those from a PWR. Because the potential for such releases from BWRs was recognized early, these reactors were

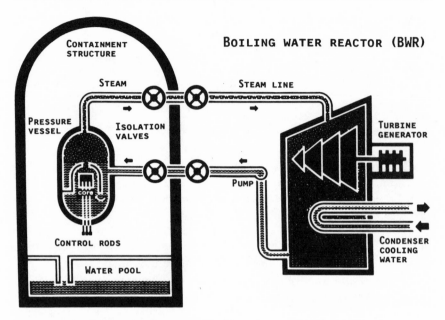

Figure 12.3   Schematic diagrams of boiling water and pressurized water
nuclear power plants

equipped with systems to capture and retain the escaping gases long
enough to permit many of them to decay. Few PWRs are equipped
with similar systems.

Table 12.2 summarizes the estimated airborne releases from representative 1,000-MWe PWRs and BWRs brought into operation since
1979. The two types of plants release about equal amounts of car-
bon-14, iodine-131, and tritium; in general, PWRs release more
krypton-85 and xenon-133 (Xe-133).

Table 12.3 shows the volumes of air required to dilute the releases
from the several types of electricity-generating plants to meet existing
U.S. federal standards for airborne contaminants in the ambient environment (EPA, 1990; NRC, 1990). The data presented are based on
the assumption that all the sulfur is released as sulfur dioxide and all
the nitrogen is released as nitrogen dioxide. In the case of coal-fired
plants, the contaminant requiring the greatest dilution would be nitrogen dioxide (NO_2). The EPA standards limit the concentration of this
pollutant in the general atmosphere to 0.053 parts per million (ppm).
The volume of air required to dilute the total annual releases of NO_2

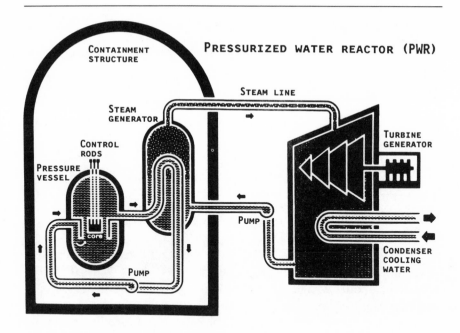

PRESSURIZED WATER REACTOR (PWR)

CONTAINMENT STRUCTURE

STEAM LINE

STEAM GENERATOR

CONTROL RODS

PRESSURE VESSEL

TURBINE GENERATOR

core

PUMP

CONDENSER COOLING WATER

PUMP

from a coal-fired plant to the EPA standard would be 4.5×10^{14} cubic meters, or about 100,000 cubic miles—obviously a tremendous volume of air. In the case of oil-fired plants, the pollutant requiring the greatest dilution is sulfur dioxide (SO_2), which the EPA limits to 0.03 ppm. The volume of air required to dilute the annual releases of SO_2 from an oil-fired power plant to an acceptable concentration would be 3×10^{14} cubic meters, or about 70,000 cubic miles. In the

Table 12.2   Annual airborne emissions from nuclear power plants
(assumed capacity 1,000 MWe)

Pollutant	Pressurized-water reactor		Boiling-water reactor	
	curies	becquerels	curies	becquerels
Krypton-85	20	7×10^{11}	—	—
Xenon-133	2,000	7×10^{13}	100	4×10^{12}
Carbon-14	10	4×10^{11}	10	4×10^{11}
Iodine-131	0.002	7×10^7	0.003	1×10^8
Tritium	150	6×10^{12}	100	4×10^{12}

Table 12.3   Annual dilution requirements for a 1,000-MWe power plant

Type of plant	Limiting pollutant	Required dilution[a]	
		m^3	mi^3
Coal	NO$_2$	4.5×10^{14}	100,000
Oil	SO$_2$	3×10^{14}	70,000
Natural gas	NO$_2$	1×10^{14}	25,000
Nuclear plant (pressurized water reactor)	Xe-133	4×10^9	1

a. Dilution requirements are approximate and are based on ambient air pollutant limits of 0.053 ppm for NO$_2$, 0.03 ppm for SO$_2$, and 2×10^{-2} Bq/cm^3 for Xe-133.

case of gas-fired plants, the pollutant requiring the greatest dilution is NO$_2$, and the volume of air required would be about 1×10^{14} cubic meters, or about 25,000 cubic miles—a significantly smaller volume than that required for a coal- or oil-fired plant of comparable size.

In the case of nuclear-powered plants, the controlling airborne pollutant is Xe-133, whose permissible ambient air concentration is 2×10^{-2} becquerels (5×10^{-7} microcuries) per cubic centimeter (ICRP, 1991a, 1991b; NRC, 1991), The volume of air needed to dilute annual releases of this radionuclide from a 1,000-MWe PWR power plant to an acceptable concentration in the ambient environment would be about 4×10^9 cubic meters, or about 1 cubic mile. This is only 0.004 percent of the volume of air needed to dilute the most critical pollutant from a comparable-sized coal-, oil-, or natural gas–fueled facility. For a BWR the volume of diluting air required would be even less.

On the basis of these data, one might conclude that a nuclear plant is far safer in terms of airborne releases than any other type. However, these calculations do not include the associated dilution requirements for the airborne gases and dusts that would be released from the tailing piles produced in conjunction with milling the uranium ore. Also not included are airborne releases that would be produced in chemically processing the spent fuel. Although chemical processing is not currently being done in the United States, it is common practice in many other countries and would need to be taken into account in those cases.

When airborne releases from various types of plants are compared, there are many factors that can influence the final numerical results (Wilson et al., 1981; Gotchy, 1987). For example, the quantity of SO_2 released from fossil-fueled plants depends on the concentration of sulfur in the fuel. The results also depend upon the environmental and public health standards being applied. Calculations of the volume of air required to dilute a given contaminant to an acceptable level assume that there is a single universally accepted concentration to which a population group can be exposed. If a higher acceptable concentration is chosen, the calculated volumes of diluting air will be lower. Another consideration is whether the standards for the permissible airborne concentrations of each pollutant are comparable. There is no assurance that each has been established on the basis of an equivalent risk (Chapter 10). Yet another factor to consider is that there are natural processes that remove pollutants such as SO_2, NO_2, and particulates from the atmosphere. Had these processes been taken into account, the quantities of diluting air required for the coal-, oil-, and gas-fired plants would have been less. Similarly, the half-life of Xe-133, the critical airborne release from a nuclear power plant, is only about 5.3 days; it too, will quickly dissipate (decay) in the ambient environment. Finally, the conclusions reached from the comparisons depend on whether the potential health impacts of the airborne contaminants are evaluated individually or collectively. In a coal-fired plant, particulates and gases are released simultaneously. If the combination of pollutants has the potential to produce synergistic effects, then the pollutants should be evaluated as a totality, not simply on the basis of the most critical individual contaminant.

Many people would want to have still other factors taken into account in an overall evaluation of the environmental and public health impact of electric power plants. In the case of fossil-fueled facilities, these include the production of acidic deposition through the release of sulfur and nitrogen compounds into the atmosphere, and the impact of the "greenhouse effect" that is postulated to result from the release of carbon dioxide (Chapter 15). In the case of nuclear-powered plants, such considerations include the long-term disposal of the associated high-level radioactive wastes (Chapter 6) and the potential for serious accidents that might release larger amounts of radionuclides into the atmosphere.

As was well illustrated by the events at Three Mile Island in Pennsylvania in 1979 and at Chernobyl in the USSR in 1986, nuclear power plant accidents can have far-reaching and long-range effects. However, it is important to keep the overall impacts of such events in perspective. The accident at Three Mile Island released only minimal amounts of radioactive materials to the environment, there were no fatalities, the total collective dose to the neighboring population was about 33 person-Sv, and more than half of the people exposed received a dose of less than 0.01 mSv. The maximum dose received by any member of the public as a result of this accident was well below 1 mSv (Rogovin, 1980).

In contrast, the accident at Chernobyl caused immediate fatalities among workers at the plant and those involved in rescue and cleanup operations, and many people in nearby areas received significant doses from airborne releases of radioactive materials. The United Nations Scientific Committee on Atomic Radiation estimates that the ultimate worldwide collective dose from this accident will be about 600,000 person-Sv (Mettler et al., 1990). About 40 percent of this dose will be received by people in the USSR, about 57 percent by people in other European countries, and about 3 percent by people elsewhere in the Northern Hemisphere. Because airborne radioactive materials do not tend to move across the Equator, people in the Southern Hemisphere will be only minimally affected; their primary source of exposure will be the consumption of imported foods that were grown in areas contaminated as a result of the accident.

About 30 percent of the collective dose was received during the first year following the Chernobyl accident; the remainder will be delivered over the next several decades. During the first year, 10–30 percent of the collective dose was from external sources, and 70–90 percent from the ingestion of radionuclides in contaminated food. After the first year, about 30 percent of the dose will be from ingestion and about 70 percent from external sources (Mettler et al., 1990).

Even though the collective-dose estimates for the Chernobyl accident appear to be high, the overall impact on the world's population was not that significant in comparison with other radiation sources to which people are exposed every day: the annual collective dose to the world's population from natural radiation sources is estimated to be about 12 million person-Sv (Mettler et al., 1990). The total projected collective dose received by the world's population as a result of the Chernobyl accident will be less than 6 percent of the collective dose being received by the same population each year from natural radiation sources. The estimated collective dose to the world's population during the first year following the Chernobyl accident was less than 2 percent of the dose received by that same population during that same year from natural background radiation sources (Mettler et al., 1990). Although no one can justify or negate the effects of the Chernobyl accident by comparing it to other sources with larger impacts, such comparisons are useful in combatting some of the unnecessary fears that many members of the public have about various radiation sources, particularly those associated with the operation of nuclear power plants.

People's fears about radiation relate not only to accidental releases from nuclear power plants but also to discharges occurring during normal operations. However, the latest epidemiological data indicate that during normal operation nuclear plants have little impact on the nearby population. On the basis of a detailed review of mortality from 16 types of cancer among people living in 107 counties near 62 major nuclear facilities in the United States, scientists at the National Cancer Institute concluded that there was no convincing evidence of any increased risk of death from living near these facilities (National Cancer Institute, 1990).

With all these factors taken into account (including the atmospheric pollution associated with the processing of spent fuel), it appears that a nuclear-powered plant has far less environmental impact than a plant fueled by oil or natural gas. All three types of facilities appear to be superior to a plant fueled with coal. If adsorption systems are used to delay the releases of radioactive gases from spent-fuel chemical reprocessing facilities, then nuclear plants remain far superior in terms of airborne releases.

Processing and Disposal of Spent Fuel

Power plants fueled by natural gas or oil have no spent-fuel disposal problems, because these fuels burn cleanly and produce essentially no ash. In coal-fired plants, however, 12–25 percent of the fuel ends up as ash. Thus, a 1,000-MWe plant would require 12–25 railroad cars for the daily removal of its ashes. Where and how these ashes are disposed is also important, since they contain many toxic compounds.

Under current operating procedures, nuclear-powered plants are shut down every 18–24 months for the removal and replacement of spent fuel. The handling and disposal of the spent fuel pose significant problems from the standpoint of radiation protection and waste disposal. Current plans are to store spent fuel at the power plant sites for a period of years (initially in water pools and later in above ground dry casks), with subsequent transport offsite for disposal in a geologic repository (Chapter 6). Where the spent fuel is chemically processed, the resulting liquid wastes will be solidified and also sent to a geologic repository for disposal. In anticipation of the associated transportation requirements, large, heavily shielded shipping casks have been designed and fabricated, and tested under a wide range of conditions. Because of the small quantities of spent fuel and solidified waste involved and the care that is to be exercised, the associated environmental and public health impacts are expected to be minimal.

Power Transmission

The type of power plant has no effect on the efficiency with which electricity is distributed to consumers. Estimates are that 12–14 percent of the electricity generated in the United States is lost during transmission. Such losses may approach 20 percent. As a result, there has been much discussion about developing new more efficient transmission systems, a promising one being the use of superconducting cables installed underground. The power losses in such a system would be less than those currently experienced in high-tension overhead power lines, and perhaps some of the questions regarding the health effects of the associated electric and magnetic fields would be avoided (Chapter 9) (Abelson, 1989). In addition, an underground system would avoid much of the environmental degradation caused by overhead lines. The swathes cut through forests and towns to accommodate overhead power lines cause extensive environmental degradation. In the United States alone there are more than 325,000 miles of overhead electric transmission lines, 10,000 miles of which operate at 750,000 volts or higher. Each mile of transmission line requires up to 100 acres of land as right-of-way (Abrahamson, 1970). If existing practices are continued, many more miles of lines will be added in the years ahead. Economics will play a major role in the installation of cables: whereas overhead lines cost about $1 million per mile to construct, underground systems are anticipated to cost as much as $10–$20 million per mile. Recent progress in developing materials that are superconductors (and can therefore transmit electricity with a minimum of losses) should enhance the potential for the use of underground systems.

The General Outlook

Urgently needed for addressing the energy question is a national energy plan, not only to address future energy needs but also to avoid repeating the errors of the past. Subsidies to the airlines, for example, have encouraged the growth of less efficient forms of transportation; lack of support of the railroad industry has discouraged the use of rail transportation. Federal support for the development of a nationwide highway system, though making road travel far safer, has led to greater use of cars, with accompanying increases in the consumption of gasoline. Another example was the shift by the railroads, immediately before and after World War II, from coal-fired steam locomotives to diesel-electric units. The Clean Air Act of 1970 also encouraged the consumption of fuels that are in limited supply, by causing industrial and power plant operators to switch from coal to natural gas and oil to meet air pollution standards. Nor has the government done anything to require changes in rate structures for natural gas and electricity, which promoted higher consumption by offering large-volume users a lower price per unit.

A national energy plan should also encourage conservation. One useful step would be to provide tax credits for the installation of insulation and solar units in dwellings. Solar units are readily available for heating homes as well as domestic water. Another step, already begun, would be to require better fuel efficiency in products ranging from automobiles to home appliances. Congress has already passed legislation that sets energy-efficiency requirements for refrigerators, hot-water heaters, and furnaces. An additional step would be to encourage the replacement of incandescent light bulbs with fluorescent lamps, which often consume as little as 25 percent as much energy. With about one-quarter of all the electricity in the United States being used for illumination, the potential for savings in this area are enormous. In fact utilities throughout the United States are already encouraging customers to adopt more efficient lighting (Lamarre, 1989).

They see conservation as preferable to the alternative—developing new electricity-generating capacity.

Household appliances might also be regulated in terms of their use of water, another limited environmental resource (Chapter 4). Conserving water will in turn reduce the energy used to purify and heat it. Examples include encouraging the use of low-flow shower heads, aerators on sink faucets, toilets that require less water to flush, and more-efficient methods of irrigating lawns, gardens, and agricultural crops.

Such conservation measures will help reduce the demand for energy, but it is unlikely that they will actually lead to a decrease in the amount consumed. Recognizing the need to conserve fossil fuels, many experts have recommended increased use of nuclear fuels. Despite its problems, this form of energy has the potential for bridging the gap until newer forms of energy, such as fusion, can be developed. Several European countries and Japan, for example, have developed energy plans that involve increasing reliance on nuclear power. One leader in this effort is France, which in 1989 generated 75 percent of its electricity with nuclear power; by 2000 it expects to be generating 90 percent of its electricity from this source. As of 1989 Belgium generated 60 percent of its electricity with nuclear power, Sweden 45 percent, Spain 38 percent, Germany 36 percent, and Japan 26 percent (U.S. Council on Energy Awareness, 1990).

The development of smaller, passively safe electric generating units (that is, units designed to limit power excursions and to shut down the reactor automatically, without the aid of external control devices) can help make the use of nuclear power more acceptable to the public. Such plants are in advanced stages of design and appear to hold promise for avoiding, or at least greatly reducing, both the probability and the consequences of accidents. Long-term growth of nuclear power, however, must rely on the use of liquid-metal fast-breeder reactors. Such units, which are being developed in countries such as France and Japan, operate at essentially atmospheric pressure and use liquid sodium as a coolant. These plants cause significantly lower radiation exposures than conventional BWR and PWR nuclear power units. Because they are more efficient, fast-breeder reactors also release less heat to the environment. Because they produce more fuel than they consume (hence the origin of the name "breeder"), fast-breeder reactors will represent an essentially unlimited energy supply.

Even with nuclear power and increased emphasis on energy conservation and the use of solar power, environmental pollution from electricity-generating plants will pose problems for many generations to come. Many of the existing coal-fueled plants are expected to have lifetimes of almost 60 years. If stringent backfitting requirements are not applied to reduce their releases of NO_2 and SO_2, these pollutants will continue to be a problem well into the next century.

However undesirable the environmental impact of electricity-generating facilities, the fact remains that electricity is essential to the quality of modern life. Better lighting reduces accidents on highways and crime in cities. Electricity is necessary to clean the air, to operate water purification facilities and sewage treatment plants, to dispose of old automobiles, and to recycle other types of solid waste. It powers radio, television, microwave ovens, computers and office equipment, and labor-saving appliances in homes. Although conservation can help reduce the overall demand for energy, the need for electricity, and thus for more power plants, will almost certainly continue to grow. The basic challenge is to educate people to use energy supplies more efficiently and to encourage the commerical sector to design, construct, and operate generating stations that function at maximum efficiency with minimal impacts on environmental health.

REFERENCES

Abelson, Philip H. 1989. "Effects of Electric and Magnetic Fields." Editorial. *Science* 245, no. 4915 (21 July), 241.

Abrahamson, Dean E. 1970. *Environmental Cost of Electric Power.* New York: Scientists' Institute for Public Information.

Anonymous. 1981. "Geothermal—Tapping the Earth's Furnace." *National Geographic,* February, pp. 66–67.

ASME. 1989. *Energy and the Environment. A General Position Paper.* New York: American Society of Mechanical Engineers.

Council on Environmental Quality. 1989. *Environmental Trends.* Washington, D.C.: Executive Office of the President.

Dickson, David. 1989. "Britain Picks Site for Wind Farm." *Science* 243, no. 4898 (24 March), 1548.

EPA. 1990. *National Air Quality and Emissions Trends Report, 1988.* Report EPA-450/4-90-002. Washington, D.C.

EPRI. 1989. *Photovoltaic Field Test Performance Assessment: 1987*. Report EPRI GS-6251. Palo Alto: Research Reports Center.

Flavin, Christopher. 1986. "Reforming the Electric Power Industry." In *State of the World,* ed. Linda Starke. New York: W. W. Norton.

General Motors Corporation. 1990. *Public Interest Report 1990,* Detroit.

Gore, Rick. 1981. "Conservation—Can We Live Better on Less?" *National Geographic,* February, pp. 34–57.

Gotchy, Reginald L. 1987. *Potential Health and Environmental Impacts Attributable to the Nuclear and Coal Fuel Cycles*. Report NUREG-0332 (final report). Washington, D.C.: U.S. Nuclear Regulatory Commission.

Hellums, W. E. 1990. "Let's All Play by the Same Rules!" Letter to the editor. *Health Physics* 58, no. 3 (March), 377.

Hubbert, M. King. 1973. *Survey of World Energy Resources*. Report of the U.S. Geographical Survey. Washington, D.C.

ICRP. 1991a. *1990 Recommendations of the International Commission on Radiological Protection*. Publication 60, Annals of the ICRP, vol. 21, no. 1–3. New York: Pergamon Press.

—— 1991b. *Annual Limits on Intake of Radionuclides by Workers Based on the 1991 Recommendations*. Publication 61, Annals of the ICRP, vol. 21, no. 4. New York: Pergamon Press.

Kirk, Don. 1989. "Bonn Launches Wind Energy Experiment." *Science* 243, no. 4898 (24 March), 1548.

Lamarre, Leslie. 1989. "Lighting the Commercial World." *EPRI Journal* 14, no. 8 (December), 4–15.

Martino, P. 1980. "LNG Risk Management." *Environmental Science & Technology* 14, no. 12, (December), 1446–54.

Mettler, F. A., W. K. Sinclair, L. Anspaugh, C. Edington, J. H. Harley, R. C. Ricks, P. B. Selby, E. W. Webster, and H. O. Wyckoff. 1990. "The 1986 and 1988 UNSCEAR Reports: Findings and Implications." *Health Physics* 58. no. 3 (March), 241–250.

National Cancer Institute. 1990. *Cancer in Populations Living near Nuclear Facilities*. Washington, D.C.: U.S. Department of Health and Human Services.

National Research Council. 1979. "Geothermal Energy." In *Energy in Transition, 1985–2010*. San Francisco: W. H. Freeman.

NRC. 1991. "Standards for Protection against Radiation." Code of Federal Regulations, Title 10, Part 20, app. B, table II.

Office of Technology Assessment. 1979. *The Direct Use of Coal*. Report OTA-E-86. Washington, D.C.

Rogovin, Mitchell. 1980. *Three Mile Island: A Report to the Commissioners and to the Public*. Vol. 1. Washington, D.C.: Special Inquiry Group, Nuclear Regulatory Commission.

Schaefer, John. 1989. "Renewable Resource Power Plants—Wind Systems." *EPRI Journal* 14, no. 5 (July/August), 49–52.

Shea, Cynthia P. 1989. "Harvesting the Wind." *World-Watch* 1, no. 2 (March–April), 12–17.

Somerville, Diana. 1989. "Whatever Happened to Solar Energy?" *American Scientist* 77, no. 4 (July–August), 328–329.

U.S. Council on Energy Awareness. 1990. "Nuclear Energy Capacity Continues Upward Trends." *INFO,* no. 254 (June), 1.

White, Gilbert F. 1988. "Environmental Effects of the High Dam at Aswan (Egypt)." *Environment* 30, no. 7 (September), 4–11 and 34–40.

Wilson, R., S. D. Colome, J. D. Spengler, and D. G. Wilson. 1981. *Health Effects of Fossil Fuel Burning.* Cambridge, Mass.: Ballinger.

Wrenn, McDonald E. 1979. "A Comparison of Occupational Human Health Costs of Energy Production: Coal and Nuclear Electric Generation." In *Energy and Health,* ed. Norman E. Breslow and Alice S. Whittemore. Philadelphia: SIAM.

13

Disaster Response

Throughout the world, natural disasters—floods, tornadoes, hurricanes, earthquakes, and volcanic eruptions—and accidents involving industrial and technological facilities (such as oil spills and accidents at nuclear power plants) have a significant impact on both people and the environment. Natural disasters alone have caused an estimated 3 million deaths worldwide over the past two decades (National Academy of Engineering, 1988). Table 13.1 summarizes the impacts of some of these events.

The economic and human costs of these disasters vary widely, depending on the concentration of population, the existence of emergency response capabilities, the area's accessibility to outside assistance, the efficiency of rescue operations, building design and construction practices, and soil conditions (Ward, 1989). Consider, for example, the human costs of three recent major earthquakes: one in Mexico City in September 1985 left 9,000 people dead, 30,000 injured, and more than 95,000 homeless; one in Soviet Armenia in December 1988 took more than 25,000 lives and left 500,000 homeless; one in northern California in October 1989 claimed only 63 lives and injured only 3,800.

Reasons for the high tolls in Mexico City and Soviet Armenia were the density of the population, inadequate building codes, lack of planning for disasters, insufficient rescue and debris-removal equipment, and lack of or heavy damage to local medical facilities (Merchant, 1986; Ward, 1989). The relatively low level of damage in California was primarily the result of strict building codes, sound construction techniques, well-organized and -rehearsed emergency response capabilities, ample communication facilities, and the increasing reliability of earthquake-forecasting techniques. The most heavily damaged area was the marina district, where buildings were constructed on landfill, which under earthquake conditions becomes like quicksand and provides essentially no support (Canby, 1990). A similar situation existed in Mexico City, where the subsoil is particularly vulnerable to earthquakes (Merchant, 1986). Delaying the response in Soviet Armenia were the mountainous terrain and the blocking of major roads by landslides.

Table 13.2 summarizes the general health effects of natural disasters. As more and more people in developing countries move into cities, where they live crowded in substandard housing and must depend on the effective functioning of the man-made environment, the human toll from disasters will continue to mount unless public authorities plan intelligently to cope with them. Recognizing the need for better capabilities in coping with natural disasters, which take especially high tolls in developing countries, the United Nations General Assembly in 1987 designated the 1990s as the International Decade for Natural Disaster Reduction. It announced five goals: (1) to improve the capacity of each country to mitigate the effects of natural disasters; (2) to devise appropriate guidelines for applying existing knowledge; (3) to foster scientific and engineering endeavors to close gaps in knowledge; (4) to disseminate new and existing information on assessment, prediction, prevention, and mitigation of natural disasters; and (5) to carry out and evaluate programs of technical assistance, technology transfer, and training (National Academy of Engineering, 1988; Pan American Health Organization, 1989).

Man-made disasters, especially in developing countries, are harder to plan for. The effects of the unanticipated system failures in the chemical plant in Bhopal, India, were compounded by several factors: public housing was located next to the plant; the release of methyl isocyanate occurred at night, delaying public awareness of the event; there was little public knowledge of the potential toxicity of emissions from the plant; and the only medical facility in the area was a small community hospital unable to cope with the needs of thousands of people (Merchant, 1986).

Few countries today provide the public with adequate information about the location of chemical manufacturing plants or the nature and quantity of chemicals being manufactured (Wasserman, 1985). Few have regulations governing transportation routes for hazardous chemi-

Table 13.1 Examples of natural and man-made disasters, 1979 and later

Type of event	Location	Date of occurrence	Impact
Natural disaster			
Volcanic eruption	Mount St. Helens, Washington	May 18, 1980	62 deaths
	Nevado del Ruiz, Colombia	November 13, 1985	25,000 deaths, thousands homeless
	Mount Pinatubo, Philippines	June–July 1991	> 500 deaths, widespread damage
Gas release	Lake Nyos, Cameroon	August 21, 1986	1,700 deaths
Earthquake	Mexico City, Mexico	September 19, 1985	9,000 deaths, 30,000 injured, 95,000 homeless
	Armenia, USSR	December 7, 1988	> 25,000 deaths, 500,000 homeless
	Northern California (Loma Prieta)	October 17, 1989	63 deaths
Hurricane	Gilbert: Jamaica, Yucatán Peninsula, northeast Mexico	September 1988	300 deaths
	Hugo: Caribbean, North Carolina, South Carolina	September 1989	18 deaths in South Carolina, many more in Caribbean
Cyclone	Bangladesh	April 30, 1991	138,000 deaths, 9 million homeless

Man-made disaster

Nuclear power plant accident	Three Mile Island, Pennsylvania	March 29, 1979	No deaths, minimal releases
	Chernobyl, USSR	April 26, 1986	31 immediate deaths, many latent cancers possible
Industrial plant accident	Methyl isocyanate release, Bhopal, India	December 2–3, 1984	2,500–5,000 deaths
Challenger space shuttle explosion	Kennedy Space Center, Florida	January 28, 1986	7 deaths
Radiation therapy machine accident	Goiânia, Brazil	September 1987	4 deaths, dozens of people contaminated
Oil-tanker spill	*Exxon Valdez*, Prince William Sound, Alaska	March 1989	11 million gallons spilled, heavy contamination
	Kharg-5, Atlantic Ocean off coast of Morocco	December 1989–January 1990	19 million gallons spilled, no contamination of coastline
	Mega Borg, Gulf of Mexico	June 1990	4 million gallons spilled
	Berge Broker, Atlantic Ocean northeast of Bermuda	November 1990	4 million gallons spilled
Oil spill (not tanker related)	Three major spills into Persian Gulf from refineries in Kuwait	January 1991	About 100 million gallons released, heavy contamination
Oil-well fires	Kuwait	February 1991–	Initially > 700 burning wells, widespread air pollution

Table 13.2 Health effects of natural disasters

Health effect	Earthquake	Hurricane, high wind	Volcanic eruption	Flood	Tidal wave, flash flood
Deaths	Many	Few	Varies	Few	Many
Severe injuries (requiring extensive medical care)	Overwhelming	Moderate	Variable	Few	Few
Increased risk of infectious disease	A potential problem in all major disasters; probability increases with overcrowding and deteriorating sanitation				
Food scarcity	Rare (may occur as a result of factors other than food shortages)	Rare	Common	Common	Common
Major population movements	Rare (may occur in heavily damaged urban areas)	Rare	Common	Common	Common

cals or systems for registering their importation, distribution, and storage. There is no centralized and coordinated international system for reporting either chemical accidents or their long-term consequences. In the United States the congressionally mandated Toxic Waste Inventory reports only toxic chemical releases to the environment; it does not require reporting of the amounts of toxic substances handled by a facility (National Research Council, 1990). Without such information, public and environmental health agencies cannot plan comprehensive responses to emergencies.

Emergency Preparedness

Technology

Technological forecasting has proved very effective in reducing the impacts of events that can be anticipated, such as volcanic eruptions. For example, the eruption of Mount St. Helens in 1980 took few lives not only because it occurred on a Sunday morning, when few loggers were in the area, and because the primary blast was toward the more sparsely populated north and northeast, but also because the National Geologic Survey had forecast the approximate time and the area likely to be affected by the release (Buist and Bernstein, 1986; Merchant, 1986).

Similarly, careful inspections can be used to alert industrial groups to impending accidents in industrial plants, and proper follow-up maintenance and repairs can be used to avert accidents. Engineering technology can also be used to design plants so that damage can be contained in the event of accidents. This approach is routinely applied in the design and operation of nuclear power plants.

Public Information and Education

Two other essential ingredients in effective preparedness for emergencies are public information and education. Informing the public about what to expect and what measures to take to avoid harm can considerably reduce the impacts of a natural disaster or industrial accident. Public officials should provide advance information about the possible effects of chemicals and about appropriate countermeasures, as well as timely warnings so that people can seek shelter or evacuate. In the event of an accident at an industrial facility, plant operators should fully inform local public and environmental health authorities about the current situation and expected developments over the next few hours and days. Table 13.3 lists several documents providing guidance on emergency planning and response.

Infrastructure

In the Americas, floods and earthquakes are the most common kinds of natural disaster. Besides disrupting transportation systems and sources of electrical power, which pose significant problems in themselves in terms of delayed rescue and medical care and food shortages, earthquakes can threaten human health on a massive scale by disrupting water supplies and the safe disposal of wastes. Water-supply and sewage-disposal facilities should be designed, built, and maintained to withstand such events.

General Emergency Response

A solid emergency plan can ensure quick and effective mobilization to respond to the immediate health-care needs of the people affected and to restore disrupted services. The plan should be clear, concise, and complete. It should also be dynamic, flexible, and subject to frequent evaluation and update. It should designate precisely who does what and when, and everyone involved should be familiar with it. Its top priority should be to provide an immediate response to the event, such as locating and providing emergency medical services to the victims, controlling fires, removing downed power lines, and controlling leaks of natural gas (Waeckerle, 1991). On a longer-range basis, the goals should be to provide health care and shelter for victims, supplemented by the restoration of important services such as a safe water supply and basic sanitation. Next in importance are arrangements to provide a safe food supply and to meet needs for personal hygiene.

In general, there are two types of emergency plans. One is national or regional in scope and defines the responsibilities and mobilization procedures of personnel in key public and environmental health departments and emergency preparedness agencies. In many cases, planning at this level includes coordination of civil defense and military services. The other level, which is local in scope, is much more

Table 13.3   Sources of information on emergency planning and response

Agency	Document
DOE	*Effectiveness of Sheltering in Buildings and Vehicles for Plutonium,* Report DOE/EH-0159T (Washington, D.C., 1990)
FEMA	*In Time of Emergency: A Citizen's Handbook,* Report H-14 (Washington, D.C., 1985)
	A Guide to Preparing Emergency Public Information Materials, Report FEMA REP-11 (Washington, D.C., 1985)
	"Federal Natural Disaster Response Plan," Draft report (Washington, D.C., 1990)
International Atomic Energy Agency	*Derived Intervention Levels for Application in Controlling Radiation Doses to the Public in the Event of a Nuclear Accident or Radiological Emergency,* Safety Series no. 81 (Vienna, 1986)
	Medical Handling of Accidentally Exposed Individuals, Safety Series no. 88 (Vienna, 1988)
	Cleanup of Large Areas Contaminated as a Result of a Nuclear Accident, Technological Report Series no. 300 (Vienna, 1989)
ICRP	*Protection of the Public in the Event of Major Radiation Accidents: Principles for Planning,* Publication 40, Annals of the ICRP (New York, 1984)
NRC	"Standard Format and Content for Emergency Plans for Fuel Cycle and Materials Facilities," Draft Regulatory Guide (Washington, D.C., 1990)
Pan American Health Organization	*Emergency Health Management after Natural Disasters* (Washington, D.C., 1985)
	Emergency Management of Environmental Health and Water Supply (Washington, D.C., 1987)
U.S. Department of Health and Human Services	*The Public Health Consequences of Disasters,* ed. M. B. Gregg (Washington, D.C., 1989)
U.S. Department of Transportation	*Emergency Response Guidebook, 1987: Guidebook for Hazardous Materials Incidents,* Report DOR P 5800.4 (Washington, D.C., 1987)

definitive and includes detailed listings of the personnel involved, their individual responsibilities during an emergency, and the range of countermeasure actions available for implementation. The local plan should be closely coordinated with the national or regional effort. Together, these two groups can provide a cadre of well-trained personnel to cope with natural disasters or industrial accidents of almost any size.

Most plans for disasters cover four phases: the time (years) before the event (the pre-event phase); the warning or alerting period, just before events that can be predicted will occur; the response phase, immediately following the event; and the recovery (rehabilitation) phase.

Pre-Event Phase

The objectives during this phase are to anticipate that accidents and disasters will occur and to plan for responding to them. Specific steps should be taken to identify all available organizational resources; make an inventory of the types and location of available supplies and equipment, including both hardware and medical supplies; identify private-sector contractors and distributors who can provide otherwise-scarce specialized personnel and equipment; review essential community and industrial facilities to identify those that may be vulnerable to a disaster; and define the responsibilities of each agency or group and establish lines of communications. In support of these activities, an emergency operations center should be designated and properly equipped.

Warning or Alerting Period

For certain types of disasters, particularly those caused by natural forces, advance warning may be available. Examples are hurricanes, tornadoes, and floods. In these cases there will be an opportunity to alert emergency planning personnel and, in fact, to have them move, where appropriate, to the emergency operations center. An important activity during this period will be to provide timely and accurate information to the media and the public about what to expect (Waeckerle, 1991). Such information should include specific details on what should be done to prepare for the event.

Response Phase

Usually fire, emergency medical, and police personnel are the first to arrive with help at the site of a major disaster. The laypeople already present will inevitably include well-meaning volunteers. Properly managed, volunteers can be helpful; otherwise they can hinder the response. Their sheer numbers alone may create a logistical problem. It is important to provide security to the affected area to assure the safety of both victims and workers. To manage these problems, the most experienced senior person should take charge, immediately surveying the area and carefully assessing the scene, the number of victims, and their injuries. This person should then relay information on the situation to the emergency operations center and make recommendations for action. Officials at the center must then determine whether the police, fire, and emergency medical personnel on-site can adequately meet the needs (Waeckerle, 1991). Details of some of the countermeasures that can be taken to protect the public from airborne chemical or radioactive material releases, such as might occur in an industrial or nuclear power accident, are discussed below.

Recovery Phase

During this phase there may be substantial numbers of injured people needing follow-up care. All survivors will require food, water, shelter, clothing, and sanitation facilities (Waeckerle, 1991). In some cases, conditions will favor rapid increases in insect and rodent populations (Pan American Health Organization, 1985). Floods, especially, promote unsanitary conditions not only through the buildup of debris and blockage of sewer systems, but also through the creation of breeding habitats for insects, such as mosquitoes, in rain and flood waters remaining on the soil, in empty receptacles, and elsewhere. To address such problems, planners should maintain up-to-date information on the distribution of vectorborne diseases in a given area and in nearby regions (Pan American Health Organization, 1982).

Nuclear Emergency Response

Planning for effective response to accidents in nuclear power plants has been remarkably thorough and complete in the developed countries. Many of the principles and procedures developed for these facilities are applicable to other types of disasters. In fact, the best emergency response plans coordinate nuclear emergency response capabilities with those for other types of industrial and natural disasters.

At the international level, the principal agencies to address this issue are the International Commission on Radiological Protection (ICRP) and the International Atomic Energy Agency (IAEA) (Table 13.3). The ICRP develops the concepts that should underlie an effective emergency plan, and the IAEA uses this information to develop definitive guidance for implementing an emergency plan. The protective measures developed by the ICRP have three goals: (1) to limit the doses to individual members of the population below the thresholds for the development of any acute effects, (2) to limit the doses that do occur so as to minimize the risks of latent cancer effects among the exposed population, and (3) to limit as far as reasonably practical the number of people receiving any doses whatever from an accident (ICRP, 1984). The protective measures taken will depend on which body organs or tissues are liable to be exposed, the level of dose that is projected if no protective or countermeasure action is taken, and the pathways by which the exposures are likely to occur.

Phases in Nuclear Response Planning

In developing protection principles for emergency planning, the ICRP has divided anticipated accidents into three phases, which correspond closely to the last three of the four phases in plans for coping with other types of disasters:

The early phase, comprising two stages: (1) the time while there is a threat of a serious release, and (2) the first few hours after commencement of a release, if the accident is not brought under control.

The intermediate phase, spanning the period from the first few hours to several days after the onset of an accident, when presumably most of the release from the facility to the atmosphere has already occurred and, unless the release has consisted primarily of the radioactive gases, there are likely to be significant amounts of radioactive material deposited on the ground. During this phase the most important routes of exposure will be: (1) external exposures arising mainly from radioactive material deposited on the ground and (2) internal exposures resulting primarily from ingestion of water and foodstuffs contaminated directly, or agricultural products such as milk that are derived from cows grazing in contaminated areas.

The recovery phase, possibly extending over a prolonged period (as in the case of the accident at the Chernobyl nuclear plant), during which decisions are made about a return to normal living conditions. The major routes of exposure during this phase will be similar to those during the intermediate phase, namely: (1) external exposures from radioactive materials persisting on the ground, on roads, and on buildings; and (2) internal exposures through the inhalation of radioactive materials resuspended from the ground or through the ingestion of contaminated foodstuffs or agricultural products grown in contaminated areas.

Countermeasures for a Nuclear Accident

Table 13.4 summarizes the countermeasures considered most appropriate for controlling population exposures at each phase of a major nuclear accident. Table 13.5 summarizes the protective measures considered appropriate to each pathway of potential population exposure. The appropriate choice of countermeasures varies with the magnitude, timing, and duration of the release of radioactive material and with local conditions such as population density, time of day, emergency resources, and transportation services. For these reasons, the selection of any countermeasure must take into account its possible impact on the public, industry, agriculture, and government. According to the U.S. Public Health Service (1962), an acceptable countermeasure must be *effective* (substantially reduce population exposures below those that would otherwise have occurred), *safe* (introduce no health risks with potentials worse than those presented by the radioactive releases), *practical* (capable of being administered at a reasonable cost and without creating legal problems), and *defined* (with no jurisdictional confusion about various agencies' responsibility and authority for applying the measure). Almost any countermeasure will carry with it health risks and social and economic disruption, depending upon when and where it is applied.

Table 13.4 Countermeasures available for each phase following an accident in a nuclear facility

Early phase	Intermediate phase	Recovery phase
Sheltering and ad hoc respiratory protection	Sheltering	
Administration of stable iodine	Administration of stable iodine	
Evacuation	Evacuation	
Control of access	Control of access	Control of access
	Relocation	Relocation
	Decontamination of people	
	Control of foodstuffs and drinking water, use of stored animal feed	Control of foodstuffs and drinking water, use of stored animal feed
	Medical care	Decontamination of land areas and buildings

Sheltering and Ad Hoc Respiratory Protection

The simplest and least disruptive of all proposed countermeasures is to have people remain indoors, much as they would for most weather-related emergencies. Sheltering can provide substantial protection in cases in which the ventilation rate of buildings is low and the time of immersion in the airborne cloud is short. The use of common household materials, such as handkerchiefs and bath towels, as breathing filters can provide effective respiratory protection against both particulates and certain volatile radionuclides. Because of their simplicity, sheltering and ad hoc respiratory protection are often proposed as viable alternatives to mass or partial evacuations, especially for people located several miles or more from the facility, and where data concerning the magnitude, duration, and direction of an airborne release are unavailable or unreliable.

Administration of Stable Iodine

If humans have a sufficient intake of stable elements, their uptake of radioactive isotopes of these same elements will be significantly reduced. This concept is used in nuclear emergency response through the administration of stable iodine to prevent uptake of radioactive iodine (I-131) by the thyroid. As Figure 13.1 indicates, however, for greatest effectiveness the stable iodine must be administered either before or very soon after exposure. Since reliable radiation monitoring data may not be available that quickly, the decision to administer stable iodine should be based on a preplanned estimate of the probable degree of contamination from an accident. Even so, administering stable iodine to the general population carries problems. If it is to be distributed after an accident has occurred, health personnel may have difficulty locating all members of the population. If it is distributed before an accident, the measure may of course later prove to have been unnecessary. In addition, the intake of stable iodine may have adverse health effects on a small percentage of the population (NCRP,

Table 13.5 Countermeasures available for each exposure pathway following an accidental airborne release from a nuclear facility

Exposure pathway	Available countermeasures
External exposure from radionuclides in airborne cloud	Sheltering, evacuation, control of access
Internal exposure from inhalation of radionuclides in cloud	Sheltering and ad hoc respiratory protection, administration of stable iodine, evacuation, control of access
External contamination from ground deposits of radionuclides	Sheltering, evacuation, control of access, decontamination
External exposure from ground deposits of radionuclides	Sheltering, evacuation, relocation, control of access, decontamination
Internal exposure from inhalation of resuspended radionuclides	Evacuation, relocation, control of access, decontamination
Internal exposure from ingestion of contaminated food and water	Control of food and water and use of stored feeds for animals

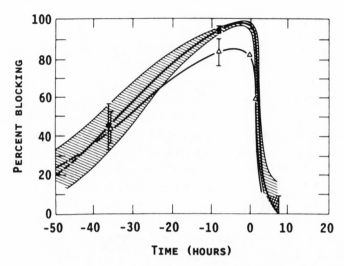

Figure 13.1   Percent of thyroid blocking afforded by the administration of 100 mg of stable iodine as a function of time before and after an assumed intake of 1 microcurie of I-131

1977). However, no health problems were reported for the thousands of people who were given stable iodine following the Chernobyl accident (Rippon, 1986).

Administration of stable iodine is clearly a sound countermeasure for emergency response personnel: police officers, firemen, physicians, radiation monitoring personnel, nurses, ambulance drivers, paramedics, and all operations personnel remaining at or returning to the facility. On the basis of information supplied by the plant operator about the magnitude of the accident, either the physician consulting for the facility or state and local public health officials can approve prompt administration of this blocking agent.

Evacuation

The feasibility of evacuation depends on the magnitude and likely duration of the release, the weather, time of day, the potential for vehicle accidents and personal injuries, the availability of transportation, the availability of suitable shelter in a "safe" area, the interval between the accident and the order to evacuate, the movement of children from schools, the movement of patients from hospitals and nursing homes, and the potential for increased uptake of releases as a result of the exertions involved (NCRP, 1977). In the case of a single-puff airborne release, it may not be possible to evacuate the neighboring population in the short time available to avoid exposure, particularly if the emergency occurs during bad weather or at an otherwise inconvenient time. In the case of a longer-term, continuous airborne release, evacuation can be very effective.

Figure 13.2 represents the protective value of evacuation procedures as a function of various conditions. As might be expected, the protective value of evacuation increases with the rapidity with which it is carried out and the distance between the airborne release and the evacuated population. Similarly, the longer the airborne cloud remains in the area, the greater the value of evacuation.

Table 13.6 summarizes the recommended upper and lower levels (based on projections of the doses that would occur if no action were taken) at which various countermeasures should be applied in the early phase of a nuclear emergency. Equally important is the estimated dose that the various protective actions will prevent. The upper dose level is the one above which countermeasures should definitely be applied; the lower dose level is the one below which countermeasures are not considered to be necessary. Another approach would be to initiate protective actions when the *dose rate* during the early phase exceeds a certain limit.

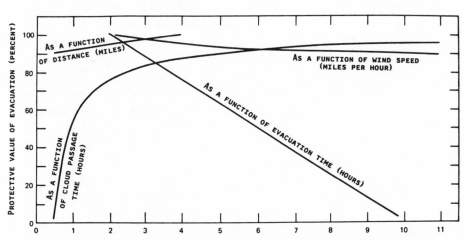

Figure 13.2   Protective value of evacuation as a function of time required for evacuation, wind speed, distance, and cloud passage time

Table 13.6 Suggested equivalent dose levels for application of
countermeasures during the early phase of a nuclear emergency

	Projected dose (mSv)[a]	
Countermeasure	Whole body	Lung, thyroid, and any single organ preferentially irradiated
Sheltering and administration of stable iodine		
Upper dose level	50	500
Lower dose level	5	50
Evacuation		
Upper dose level	500	5,000
Lower dose level	50	500

a. The suggested levels are based on projections of the doses if no protective actions were taken.

Control of Foodstuffs

MILK AND DAIRY PRODUCTS

Since the potential for internal exposure from the consumption of contaminated milk and dairy products may extend for many miles from the accident site, and since the longer-range exposure through this pathway may be 400–700 times greater than through inhalation, immediate protective action is essential. Figure 13.3 shows how rapidly radioactive materials appear in milk following a single airborne release with subsequent contamination of pasture grass. Table 13.7 lists the various countermeasures and their effectiveness in preventing radionuclide contamination of milk. Table 13.8 shows the intakes that can be avoided for four different radionuclides as a function of the time at which a specific countermeasure—that is, removing the cows from contaminated pasture—is applied.

To protect people from the intake of radionuclides via the milk pathway following a major release from a nuclear facility, a predetermined emergency communications plan must be set in motion promptly to alert dairy farmers in areas affected by the accidental release. Immediately transferring cows from outdoor pasture to stored feed will largely prevent the contamination of their milk. To be effective, such action must include placing harvested grain, hay, or silage under protective cover before the release, or removing the outer layers from exposed bales before feeding the hay to the cows.

State and local sanitarians or milk control specialists should be immediately assigned to milk distribution centers or processing plants that are likely to receive milk from contaminated farms. They should:

Establish immediate liaison with the milk industry and the officials responsible for taking protective actions

Identify the dairy farms in the affected areas shipping milk to the plant and determine if the cows on those farms are on stored feed

Provide drivers of bulk milk tankers with guidelines and requirements covering protective actions in effect and instruct them not

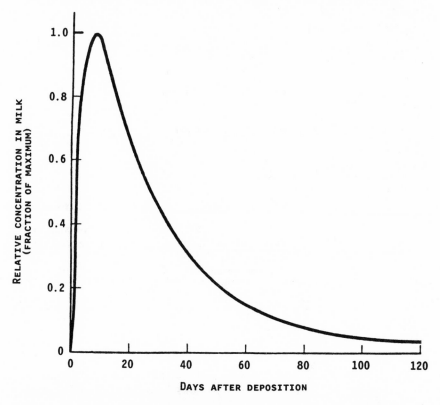

Figure 13.3   Concentration of radionuclides in milk as a function of time following a single deposition on pasture

Table 13.7 Effectiveness of countermeasures that can be applied to the pasture-milk-human pathway following an airborne release of radioactive material

Action	Radionuclides involved	Effectiveness of action (%)
For cows		
Provide alternate source of un-contaminated feed	I-131, Sr-89, Sr-90 Cs-137	90
Add stable iodine to feed ration	I-131	< 90
Add stable calcium to feed ration	Sr-89, Sr-90	< 90
Add binders to feed ration	Cs-137, Sr-89, Sr-90	< 90
Substitute water from uncon-taminated source	Cs-137, Sr-89, Sr-90	< 90
For milk		
Condemn milk supplies	I-131, Sr-89, Sr-90, Cs-137	90
Divert fresh milk to processed milk products	I-131, Sr-89	90
Process but store for later sale	I-131	90
	Sr-90, Cs-137	< 90
Remove radionuclides	I-131, Sr-89, Sr-90, Cs-137	90

Table 13.8 Intake avoided via milk pathway as a function of time of initiation of protective actions following an accidental single airborne release of radioactive material[a]

Projected intake avoided (%)	Iodine-131 (days)	Strontium-89 (days)	Strontium-90 (days)	Cesium-137 (days)
50	5–7	13	17	14
75	2–4	6	7	5
90	< 1	2	2	2

a. Days after initial contamination of pasture when cows are assumed to have been shifted to uncontaminated feed.

to accept milk from farmers having cows on outdoor pasture in the affected areas

Help the milk industry establish a procedure for collecting contaminated milk in excess of acceptable levels for diversion to a nonfluid milk processing plant

Ensure that processed milk products containing unacceptable levels are stored to await decay of radioiodine and are monitored before release for public consumption

Collect representative samples of raw milk and finished products as needed and based upon laboratory capacity

Radioiodine (I-131). In addition to removing cows from contaminated pasture, countermeasures effective in limiting human intake of radioiodine through milk include placing children, lactating mothers, and pregnant women on evaporated milk or powdered dry skim milk, and diverting fresh milk to products such as butter, cheese, or ice cream to permit decay of this short-lived radionuclide. If fresh milk supplies are also likely to be contaminated with longer-lived radionuclides, such as strontium-90, diversion to other products will not be effective.

Radiostrontium (Sr-89 and Sr-90). Placing cows on stored (uncontaminated) feed will also be helpful in reducing contamination of milk with short-lived strontium-89. Countermeasures that can be used to control contamination of milk by the longer-lived strontium-90 include treating the soil on which pasture grass is grown and altering the cows' diet. Because the chemical behavior of strontium and calcium is similar, adding lime (calcium hydroxide) to the soil will reduce the concentration of Sr-90 in pasture grass by 50–75 percent. A similar reduction will be observed in the concentrations of Sr-90 in milk. Adding stable calcium to cows' feed will reduce Sr-90 concentrations in milk by as much as 75 percent. On the other hand, supplementing diets with stable strontium alone has not proved effective, because concentrations of Sr-90 in milk are affected by the combined level of stable strontium and calcium in the cow's system, not by the level of either one alone (U.S. Public Health Service, 1962).

Similarly, attempts to remove strontium-90 from fresh fluid milk by ion-exchange processes have not proved feasible on a commercial basis (U.S. Public Health Service, 1961). Other processes that might be considered include deep-plowing to reduce the uptake of strontium-90 by shallow-rooted crops, removal of several inches of surface soil before planting additional crops, and switching to other crops, such as those with a low calcium-to-caloric ratio.

Radiocesium (Cs-137). The control of this radionuclide has many of the same difficulties associated with Sr-90. Because Cs-137 is long-lived, it cannot be controlled over extensive periods by placing cows on stored feed or by diverting fresh milk to products such as butter. Fortunately, Cs-137 tends to be tightly bound in claylike soils and thus becomes unavailable for uptake by pasture grass (Federal Radiation Council, 1965). However, in areas where sandy soils predominate, uptake of Cs-137 by pasture grass can be substantial.

AGRICULTURAL PRODUCTS AND DRINKING WATER

The major crops of concern during immediate response to an accidental airborne release of radioactive material will be those that grow aboveground (such as lettuce and cabbage), since they will be directly exposed to any radioactive fallout. These products may have to be condemned and destroyed if significant contamination is detected. Crops that grow underground, such as carrots, beets, and potatoes, will pose no problem until enough time has passed for the radioactive material to gain access to them via root uptake through the soil. Such vegetables that have already been harvested and been directly contaminated by airborne deposition can be decontaminated by washing with clean water. Similarly, fruit such as oranges and bananas can be made acceptable for human consumption simply by removing the outer peel.

On farmland that has suffered extensive radionuclide contamination, the soil must be treated so that contamination is reduced to safe levels. Idling, or nonuse, for a specific period is one strategy. Another is deep-plowing to move radioactive material below the root level, prevent the plants from taking up contaminated nutrients, and allow radionuclides to decay. Highly contaminated soil may have to be removed and disposed of elsewhere. In some circumstances alternative crops, such as cotton and flax, which would contribute no radioactive material to the diet, can be grown in place of food crops.

Covered wells and underground sources of drinking water will probably not be contaminated. Any radioactive material deposited on the soil will take a long time to travel to underground sources, and significant contamination of those sources is highly unlikely. For contaminated surface water, normal treatment processes (such as coagulation and filtration; Chapter 4) are very effective in removing particulates (Oak Ridge National Laboratory, 1959). However, removal of dissolved radionuclides will require treatment with different processes, such as ion exchange or evaporation. Even evaporation will not remove volatile radionuclides. Standard methods for monitoring public drinking-water supplies have been published (Greenberg, Trussell, and Clesceri, 1985), and many water purification facilities in larger U.S. cities have the laboratory and radiation counting equipment necessary to carry out this monitoring.

Table 13.9 lists the upper and lower dose levels for application of countermeasures for relocation and control of foodstuffs. In this case, the levels are based on projections of the doses during the first year following an accident. Establishment of these levels and the ones presented in Table 13.6 obviously depends on a wide range of circumstances.

The General Outlook

Planning to cope with natural and man-made disasters is an enormous undertaking. Government officials at all levels must work together to devise a comprehensive strategy to meet the multitude of needs created by the associated casualties, major property damage, and disruption of services. Because the same principles for response apply to a wide range of natural disasters and man-made accidents, the most successful plans assign a single group responsibility for responding to all such emergencies.

Experience has shown that dividing disasters into temporal phases can be useful in developing a sound emergency response. Those planning for responses to nuclear power plant accidents have extended this concept, adding spatial considerations. Thus, the primary protective measure for people living within one or two miles of a plant is evacuation; for those living farther away, the primary countermeasures are sheltering and respiratory protection. Such an approach will generally provide greater protection with far less disruption of off-site populations than would mass evacuation of all potentially affected population groups.

Most natural disasters, such as earthquakes, floods, tornadoes, and hurricanes, leave buildings, bridges, and roads heavily damaged. Repair and replacement are costly, but at least techniques for restoration

Table 13.9   Suggested equivalent dose levels for application
of countermeasures during the intermediate phase
of a nuclear emergency

Countermeasure	Projected equivalent dose (mSv) in first year	
	Whole body	Individual organs preferentially irradiated
Control of foodstuffs		
Upper dose level	50	500
Lower dose level	5	50
Relocation		
Upper dose level	500	Not anticipated
Lower dose level	50	Not anticipated

exist. For disasters such as oil spills and major chemical or radioactive material releases, which may involve extensive contamination of water, land, or facilities, there are as yet no simple techniques available for removing or stabilizing the contamination and restoring such areas to a usable state. A promising solution is bioremediation, through which microorganisms—individual and combinations of natural fungi and bacteria, as well as new microbes developed through genetic engineering—supplemented by nutrients, are introduced into soil or water to stabilize toxic materials (Douglas, 1988). Though in its infancy, bioremediation is being used more and more; a salient example is the use of certain types of bacteria to convert spilled crude oil into nontoxic material (Holden, 1990).

Although certain aspects of natural disasters are outside the realm of human control, there is much that can be done to reduce both the numbers and effects of man-made disasters. As in the case of other environmental hazards, assurance that adequate attention is being paid to all avenues for control requires a systems approach. In this regard, it is worth noting that the matrix method (Haddon, 1970) that has been so successfully applied to the control of vehicular accidents (Chapter 8) is equally applicable to nuclear power plant accidents. Like vehicular accidents, nuclear power plant accidents can be divided into pre-event, event, and post-event phases. The crucial factors to consider are the plant operator, the nuclear plant itself, and the environment or site. Following the analogy of vehicular accidents, steps that can be taken during the pre-event stage with respect to plant operators include proper screening and thorough training; steps that can be taken to protect operators during an event include shielded control rooms with self-contained air-cleaning systems; steps that can be taken after the event include decontamination and the provision of medical care, if needed. Proper design, construction, maintenance, and operation will help assure that the plant is not subject to an accident; providing the reactor with a containment will prevent the release of radioactive material should an accident occur; coolant sprays in containment will reduce pressure and remove airborne radioactive materials after an accident has occurred, and a passive cool-down system will remove residual decay heat from the reactor core. Steps that can be taken with respect to the environment and protection of the public during the pre-event phase include siting the plant in areas of low population density and away from seismic hazards; steps that can be taken during an accident include having instrumentation to provide meteorological data for projecting off-site doses and determining the best protective measures to recommend. Steps that can be taken in the environment to assure proper protection of the public after the accident has occurred include sheltering and respiratory protection, and having ample vehicles to evacuate close-in populations, as well as reception centers for housing and feeding them.

References

Buist, A. S., and R. S. Bernstein, eds. 1986. "Health Effects of Volcanoes: An Approach to Evaluating the Health Effects of an Environmental Hazard." *American Journal of Public Health,* supp. to vol. 76 (March).

Canby, Thomas Y. 1990. "Earthquake—Prelude to the Big One." *National Geographic* 177, no. 5 (May), 76–105.

Douglas, John. 1988. "Cleaning Up with Biotechnology." *EPRI Journal* 13, no. 6 (September), 14–21.

Federal Radiation Council. 1965. *Background Material for the Development of Radiation Protection Standards: Protective Action Guides for Strontium-89, Strontium-90, and Cesium-137.* Report no. 7. Washington, D.C.

Greenberg, A. E., R. R. Trussell, and L. C. Clesceri, eds. 1985. *Standard Methods for the Examination of Water and Wastewater*. 16th ed. Washington, D.C.: American Public Health Association.

Haddon, William. 1970. "On the Escape of Tigers: An Ecologic Note." *American Journal of Public Health* 60, no. 12 (December), 2229–34.

Holden, Constance. 1990. "Gulf Slick a Free Lunch for Bacteria." *Science* 249, no. 4965 (13 July), 120.

ICRP. 1984. *Protection of the Public in the Event of Major Radiation Accidents*. Publication 40, Annals of the ICRP, vol. 14, no. 2. New York: Pergamon Press.

Merchant, J. A. 1986. "Preparing for Disaster." Editorial. *American Journal of Public Health* 76, no. 3 (March), 233–235.

National Academy of Engineering, Advisory Committee on International Decade of Hazard Reduction. 1988. *Confronting Natural Disasters: An International Decade for Natural Hazard Reduction*. Washington, D.C.

National Research Council. 1990. "Tracking Toxicants." *NewsReport* 40, no. 6 (June), 14–15.

NCRP. 1977. *Protection of the Thyroid Gland in the Event of Releases of Radioiodine*. Report no. 55. Bethesda, Md.

Oak Ridge National Laboratory. 1959. *Report of the Joint Program of Studies on the Decontamination of Radioactive Waters*. Report ORNL-2557. Oak Ridge, Tenn.

Pan American Health Organization. 1982. *Emergency Vector Control after Natural Disaster*. Washington, D.C.

———— 1985. *Emergency Health Management after Natural Disaster*. Washington, D.C.

———— 1989. *Disaster Preparedness in the Americas*, no. 37 (January).

Rippon, Simon. 1986. "Chernobyl: The Soviet Report." *Nuclear News* 29, no. 13 (October), 59–66.

U.S. Public Health Service. 1961. *Report on the Removal of Radiostrontium from Milk*. Washington, D.C.: U.S. Department of Health, Education and Welfare.

———— 1962. *Radioactive Contamination of the Environment: Public Health Action*. Washington, D.C.: National Advisory Committee on Radiation, U.S. Department of Health, Education and Welfare.

Waeckerle, Joseph F. 1991. "Disaster Planning and Response." *New England Journal of Medicine* 324, no. 12 (21 March), 815–821.

Ward, Kaari, ed. 1989. *Great Disasters: Dramatic True Stories of Nature's Awesome Powers*. Pleasantville, N.Y.: Reader's Digest Association.

Wasserman, Ellen. 1985. "Technological Disasters in the Americas: A Public Health Challenge." *WHO Chronicle* 39, no. 3, pp. 95–97.

14

A Macroscopic View

Many of our environmental problems, such as air and water pollution, solid waste, and food contamination, are consequences of large-scale cultural patterns. Some are the net result of millions of people making individual decisions; others are the outcome of actions by a small number of people with key decision-making powers in industry, government, and academia. Although many of these problems are local, ozone depletion, the greenhouse effect, acidic deposition, and associated potential climatic changes have global implications. Solving these problems will require cutting across the divides of national jurisdictions. Also required will be a shift in focus from protection and restoration to planning and prevention.

Our global problems appear to reflect three major trends (Speth, 1989). First, as a result of a threefold increase in the world's population and a twentyfold increase in the values of goods produced since 1900, the quantity of pollutants being generated has also significantly increased. Second, there has been a shift from the use of natural products to the production and use of synthetic chemicals. For example, 1 billion pounds of synthetic pesticides are used every year in the United States. Many of these chemicals have proved to be highly toxic, and some persist and accumulate in biological sytems and in the atmosphere. Third, as a result of expanded technological capabilities and, in some cases, exports of hazardous technologies from developed to developing countries, the developing countries have become as polluted as the developed ones.

There is no consensus on how to solve these increasingly difficult environmental problems. An international treaty in 1987, the Montreal Protocol on Substances That Deplete the Ozone Layer, did establish ways to reduce the use of chlorofluorocarbons and other chemicals that destroy stratospheric ozone, but not all nations have signed it. Scientific questions remain about the impacts of the greenhouse gases and the potential for global warming (Fri, 1989), and about the discharges of pollutants that lead to acidic deposition.

Ozone Depletion

Chlorofluorocarbons (CFCs) have been widely used over the past 60 years as refrigerants in household appliances and air conditioners, as industrial solvents, as blowing agents in manufacturing foam products, and as propellants for aerosol sprays. As their name implies, these chemical compounds consist of chlorine, fluorine, and carbon atoms. Some CFCs also include hydrogen atoms. When released into the air, CFCs mix with other compounds and rise slowly into the stratosphere, where they may remain for years. In the stratosphere, ultraviolet (UV) radiation destroys the CFC molecules, releasing very reactive chlorine atoms. These, in turn, react with ozone, converting it into normal oxygen. A single CFC molecule can destroy tens of thousands of molecules of ozone. Table 14.1 summarizes the use and emission profiles of chemicals that result in destruction of the ozone layer.

Although ozone is considered a pollutant when it is near the ground, in the stratosphere it shields the earth's surface from UV radiation. The harmful effects of excess UV radiation include increased skin cancers and cataracts, lower crop yields, and damage to materials such as vinyl plastics (Chapter 9).

Everyone agrees on the need to reduce the production of CFCs. In fact, in 1990 the Montreal Protocol was revised to phase out CFC production by the year 2000. This step reinforces the urgency of developing alternative chemicals or technologies. CFCs are nontoxic and have significantly better refrigeration properties than any of the alternatives currently being considered as replacements. They also require little energy to produce. Although the processes required to manufacture alternatives will apparently be more complicated than existing CFC processes, a range of substitutes is now being evaluated, and significant research and development are under way to commercialize them. Also encouraging is the fact that several CFC producers have formed consortia to share costs and expedite the processes required for testing the toxicity of these new compounds, and to evaluate their

Table 14.1 Use and emission profiles of chemicals that result in destruction of the ozone layer, 1985

Chemical	Emissions (1000s of tons)	Atmospheric lifetime[a] (years)	Use	Annual growth rate (%)	Share of contribution to depletion (%)
CFC-12	454	139	Air conditioning, refrigeration, aerosols, foams	5	45
CFC-11	262	76	Foams, aerosols, refrigeration	5	26
CFC-113	152	92	Solvents	10	12
Carbon tetrachloride	73	67	Solvents	1	8
Methyl chloroform	522	8	Solvents	7	5
Halon 1301	3	101	Fire extinguishers	n.a.	4
Halon 1211	79	22	Refrigeration, foams	11	0

a. Time it takes for 63% of the chemical to be washed out of the atmosphere.

effects and those of their degradation products on the environment (Manzer, 1990).

Acidic Deposition

Some airborne pollutants, after being discharged by electric power plants, industrial installations, and automobiles, are chemically transformed into acid compounds. Although some of these compounds remain in solid form, the nitrogen oxides are transformed into nitric acid, and the sulfur oxides, such as sulfur dioxide (SO_2), are transformed into sulfuric acid. As a result of these transformations, the concentration of acid compounds in the atmosphere of the northeastern United States and eastern Canada is significantly higher than it was 30 years ago. The deposition of these compounds, either dry or as nitric or sulfuric acid in rain or snow, is imposing an unprecedented and alarming burden on forests, streams, and lakes in these areas. Prevention of further ecosystem damage will require a substantial reduction in the discharges of these pollutants, especially SO_2 (Harrington, 1988).

The principal measures for controlling acidic deposition and its effects are (1) to reduce the discharges of sulfur and nitrogen oxides to the atmosphere and (2) to treat sensitive ecosystems to make them less susceptible to damage. At present, experts believe that SO_2 accounts for about two-thirds of the total acidic deposition in the northeastern United States and eastern Canada; nitrogen oxides account for the rest. In acknowledgment of this fact, the Clean Air Act Amendments of 1990 mandated a 50 percent reduction by the year 2,000 in releases of SO_2 from coal-fired plants in the Midwest. To control acidic deposition in the southwestern United States, including cities such as Los Angeles, where nitrogen oxide emissions from autmobiles are a principal source, the Clean Air Act Amendments require increased controls on emissions from automobiles. Since some of the mandated emission standards may be difficult to meet with current designs, automobile manufacturers are actively exploring alternative fuels and electric units. Although no remedial actions have been developed for treating terrestrial ecosystems that have been damaged by acidic deposition, it is common practice today to add lime to lakes to increase their ability to absorb the resulting acidity. However, many uncertainties remain about the cost-effectiveness and environmental consequences of this procedure (Harrington, 1988).

The Greenhouse Effect

Today there is increasing anxiety that chemical compounds, primarily carbon dioxide (CO_2), methane, and CFCs, are causing a warming of the earth. These gases are transparent to shortwave electromagnetic radiation reaching the earth from the sun, but they absorb this radiation when it is reflected back from the earth at reduced energy into the atmosphere. In theory, increasing the concentration of these gases in the atmosphere will cause the temperature near the surface of the earth to increase, much like a greenhouse. Although there is still controversy about the degree of warming that is actually occurring, what is now known appears to be sufficient to warrant serious attention to this problem.

Atmospheric concentrations of CO_2 are increasing by about 0.4 percent per year, and overall concentrations have increased by 25 percent in the last century. In fact the concentrations today are higher than at any time during the past 160,000 years (Warrick and Jones, 1988). Once released into the atmosphere, CO_2 can be removed by several processes. Some is absorbed into the oceans; some is absorbed by trees and other vegetation. However, the exact nature of these processes is not known. Further complicating the situation are the complexities and uncertainties of the mathematical models necessary for predicting the trends and consequences of the greenhouse effect. Nonetheless, such computations suggest that the earth may be warming faster than ever before. The consequences, which include changes in rainfall patterns and in levels of the oceans, could be serious for some parts of the world. Some scientists predict a rise of as much as one meter in the level of the oceans over the next century. Such a change could flood as much as 7,000 square miles of land in the United States (Titus, 1989). Similar problems would exist for the Netherlands and Bangladesh. In central Europe, higher temperatures and the potential for extended droughts could turn fertile farmlands into deserts. Some experts estimate that even if global warming abruptly stopped in the year 2030, sea levels would continue to rise for perhaps another 1,000 years.

For the past 200 years, the cumulative addition of CO_2 to the atmosphere has come in approximately equal proportions from deforestation and combustion of fossil fuel. Today combustion accounts for about 80 percent of annual CO_2 emissions. Thus, CO_2 production is closely related to energy usage. Although the industrialized nations, most particularly the United States and the Soviet Union, have been the major contributors of CO_2 in the past, today Brazil, China, and India also rank as major global warmers. In 1987, a year of intense land clearing by fire in the Amazon Valley, Brazil accounted for more CO_2 emissions than the United States. Projections are that by the year 2025 the developing nations will be emitting four times as much CO_2 as the developed world now produces (World Resources Institute, 1990).

During the past 200 years, atmospheric concentrations of methane have approximately doubled as a result of a surge in worldwide population and in rice farming and animal husbandry. Methane is produced by the decomposition of plant matter in the stomachs of cattle and is released as flatulence; decaying vegetation in wet rice paddies also produces large quantities of this gas. Another source is biomass burning related to agricultural expansion. India, through its production of methane, now ranks among the top five producers of greenhouse gases. Currently, methane concentrations in the atmosphere are increasing at a rate of about 1 percent per year (Warrick and Jones, 1988).

The ideal solution would be to slow the rate of increase of atmospheric concentrations of the greenhouse gases. However, it will be extremely difficult to reconcile such control measures with the needs of the world's burgeoning population. This environmental problem, like that of ozone depletion, can be solved only through international cooperation. One major step for control would be to promote the use of energy sources, such as solar and nuclear power, that do not produce CO_2.

Deforestation

At one time forests covered 70 percent of the land area of the world. Today this is no longer the case. India has lost two-thirds of its forests since 1900. The contiguous United States has lost 90 percent of its forests since 1620. Worldwide, satellite sensing shows that tropical rain forests are being destroyed at a rate of 40–50 million acres (60,000–75,000 square miles) per year (World Resources Institute, 1990). If current trends continue, most of the forests of the Amazon will be lost by the year 2000 (Table 14.2).

The cutting and hauling of trees from a forest is equivalent to removing the essential nutrients and topsoil. Water and nutrient cycles

Table 14.2   Loss of tropical rain forests, 1991

Forest	Original area (1000s of acres)	Remaining area (1000s of acres)	% loss
Tropical Andes	25,000	8,600	66
Atlantic forest, Brazil	247,000	4,940	98
Madagascar	15,314	2,470	84
Indonesia	301,340	130,910	57
Philippines	61,750	1,976	97
Total	650,404	148,896	77

are destabilized, and the soil itself is left unprotected from flooding and erosion. The resulting sharp decline in soil fertility reduces agricultural productivity. Without the moisture retention capability provided by the trees, floods occur. Without the trees themselves, there is less transpiration of moisture into the air and less rainfall in neighboring areas, and the slow release of water from the forests to streams during dry periods ceases. This leads to droughts, with the net result being cycles of drought and floods, and, finally, deserts. Constructing dams to control the water can cause a multitude of other public and environmental health problems (Council on Environmental Quality, 1981) (Chapter 12).

With 60 percent of the people in the world still using wood for cooking, and with businesses relying on forest resources for timber products, tobacco curing, and other industrial applications, additional deforestation is inevitable. Intensified management of the remaining forests to raise yields and an increase in the areas devoted to timber plantations will have both positive and negative effects on the environment. Well-managed plantations and production forests can reduce the harvesting of trees from natural forests, but plantation forests are biologically less diverse, are poorer habitats for native animals, and, in some instances, may be inferior in retaining the water and in conserving the soil. In addition, successful operation of such forests may require the use of pesticides, herbicides, and energy-intensive fertilizers (Council on Environmental Quality, 1981).

The destruction of forests may be leading to changes in the global climate. Some people estimate that as much as half of the carbon in the world's biomass may be stored in forests. As a result deforestation reduces the earth's capacity to absorb carbon dioxide from the atmosphere, and it also significantly reduces biotic diversity. According to current estimates, there are 3–10 million species of flora and fauna on earth. Their diversity provides an index of the ecological health of the planet. Until the twentieth century, very few species were extinguished as a result of human activities; in recent years, however, the number has increased significantly. Some groups estimate that as many as 3 species are disappearing every day, and this rate appears to be accelerating. If this trend continues, by the year 2000 as many as 20 percent of the species now on earth could be extinct (Council on Environmental Quality, 1981).

Extinction is an irreversible process. Lost with these plants and animals will be critical genetic information and biotic resources, including natural chemical compounds that could have useful medical applications. Examples of benefits already derived from exotic animals and plants include a drug to treat high blood pressure, using venom from the pit viper in Brazil; the use of genes from tropical tomatoes to increase the density of U.S. tomatoes, with added profits to catsup manufacturers; the potential use of natural protein from wild Mexican beans to repel insects without poisoning the soil or water; and the use of high-yield African plants, rather than trees, as a source of pulp for paper (Linden, 1989). One scientist has likened the current reduction of biodiversity to "burning a library before the books have been read" (Bertrand, 1990).

Steps that can be taken to counteract the loss of forests include programs for reforestation, such as the one in Brazil, which offers tax incentives to industry to encourage the planting of trees; restrictions on land clearing, based on soil capability studies; better management of present rangelands, including controls on grazing and improvement of pasture; better management of existing forest resources; the use of more-efficient wood cooking stoves; and development of biogas and solar stoves to replace wood burners (Council on Environmental Quality, 1981).

Loss of Topsoil

Accelerated erosion occurs where human activity disrupts the plant cover that usually protects the soil. Poor farming techniques such as deep-plowing, followed by wind and water erosion, are major causes of topsoil losses. In the United States alone, 1.7 billion tons of topsoil are lost annually, 300 million of which wind up in the Gulf of Mexico (AMA, 1990). Also contributing to this problem is urban/suburban sprawl, through which farmlands with acres of the world's richest topsoil are being covered by asphalt parking lots, housing developments, and shopping malls.

Soil loss by erosion involves more than just depletion of the topsoil. Soil washing off cropland, pasture, or forest land ends up in surface water, in the air, or on other lands. Sediment in water bodies causes turbidity, silting, and deterioration of aquatic habitats, decreases storage capacity in lakes and reservoirs, and interferes with water distribution systems. Fertilizers, pesticides, and salts in eroded sediments reduce water quality. Soil particles blown by wind can cause dust storms that physically damage crops and buildings. Windblown particles can also contribute in a major way to air pollution, exacerbating respiratory ailments and impairing vision (Council on Environmental Quality, 1989).

Once removed, topsoil requires hundreds to thousands of years for regeneration. Without appropriate conservation practices, farming, livestock grazing, logging, and other activities will continue to cause soil erosion. Among the most successful techniques for erosion control are various forms of conservation tillage in which a residue from a previous crop is left in the field, contour plowing, maintenance of vegetative buffer strips between fields and along waterways, planting highly erodible soils with permanent trees or grass cover, and keeping a vegetative cover on idle land (Council on Environmental Quality, 1989).

Destruction of Wetlands

Wetlands include tidal marshes, swamp forests, peat bogs, prairie potholes, and wet meadows. They are the most highly biologically productive ecosystems in the world. Wetlands serve as nurseries and feeding grounds for a range of commercial fish species, as nesting and feeding grounds for waterfowl and migratory birds, and as a habitat for many forms of other animal life (otters, turtles, frogs, snakes, and insects). In addition, wetlands trap nutrients and sediments; purify water by removing coliform bacteria, heavy metals, and toxic chemicals; provide flood protection by slowing and storing water; and anchor shorelines and provide erosion protection.

As of 1980, more than 100 million acres of wetlands in the contiguous United States had been drained, cleared, or filled (Canby, 1980). In 1950–1970 alone, 10 million acres of wetlands were lost. Although most of those lands were converted to agricultural use, urban development accounted for approximately 10 percent of this loss; another 5 percent were lost to suburban residential developments, highways, airports, industrial facilities, and marinas (Council on Environmental Quality, 1989).

Section 404 of the Federal Water Pollution Control Act of 1972 assigned the U.S. Army Corps of Engineers responsibility for defining and supervising wetlands. Initially, the Corps's regulations applied only to navigable waterways and their adjacent wetlands. In 1976 the final regulations expanded the definition of wetlands to include lands adjacent not only to navigable waterways and their tributaries but also to other rivers and streams and to natural lakes of at least 5 acres (O'Connor, 1977). As a result of these and other efforts, 104 million acres (some 5 percent of the contiguous 48 states) are now officially designated as wetlands. Three-quarters of these lands are privately owned. Owing to a flurry of criticism by land owners, however, the government recently narrowed its definition of wetlands, to exclude lands that are flooded only on a periodic basis. Such a change will now permit these lands to be converted to other uses (Carpenter, 1991). No one questions the value of wetlands as an environmental resource. The major challenge is to balance human needs and desires with the preservation of the environment.

The General Outlook

In addition to global environmental health problems, each country confronts a host of local challenges. To meet them successfully, policymakers need to seek out the root causes of these problems wherever possible and maintain perspective in setting priorities for addressing them.

Prevention or control of environmental problems requires knowledge, technology, and the will and incentive to use them. For example, industrialists and industrial engineers must learn to incorporate sound environmental thinking in the initial selection and design of manufacturing processes and products (National Academy of Engineering, 1989). Pollution controls should be designed into industrial equipment, not added on later.

Our society as a whole needs to develop a proactive attitude in dealing with environmental problems, instead of merely reacting when a crisis develops. Societal behavior can change when enough people become aware of environmental problems and act, both as individuals and through their elected representatives in government. The American Medical Association, in its policy statement *Stewardship of the Environment,* suggests that the United States should play a leading role in effecting change (1989, p. 2):

> The U.S. and the world at large appear to be facing environmental threats of unprecedented proportions, and scientists, environmental activists, health professionals, politicians and world leaders are beginning to realize the need for changes in societal behavior (i.e., human behavior as well as the conduct of business and industry) as a means of forestalling these potential threats. Societal changes must be initiated worldwide if they are to have any significant effect overall. However, their implementation will need a model, most suitably a national model . . . The U. S. could well become a model for environmental stewardship if a grassroots movement were to develop to encourage and endorse a protective and nurturing philosophy towards the environment at both the personal and societal levels.

Accomplishing these objectives will require action on several fronts, one of the most important of which is education. According to the EPA's National Advisory Council on Environmental Policy and Technology, the most productive such effort will be directed to young people, and it should be designed to inculcate environmental values during primary and secondary school (EPA, 1989). Even then, such a program can be effective only if it has the support of the entire community—schools, churches, business and industry, trade associations and professional groups, advertising and news media, and government at all levels (AMA, 1989).

In spite of what may often seem an insurmountable task, progress is being made. About 80 percent of Americans are very concerned about their environment, especially air and water quality; about half to two-thirds are also worried about the greenhouse effect, ozone depletion, and hazardous substances at home and at work (Somerville, 1989). The will is there; the knowledge and technology continue to evolve. The primary need is the leadership to marshal existing support and to set priorities for action.

Progress in controlling environmental degradation on a global scale requires the commitment and support of every nation in the world, individually and collectively. Although the Montreal Protocol on ozone depletion may not furnish an exact model for addressing all global issues, it has provided insights on a process for negotiating solutions to these types of problems. Hopefully, it will be possible over the next few years to develop multilateral and international agreements on other issues having worldwide impacts, including global warming, deforestation, energy conservation, and a wider exchange of data on protecting the environment (Morrisette, 1990). International meetings, such as the 1992 United Nations Conference on Environment and Development, are providing excellent forums for addressing such issues.

REFERENCES

AMA, Council on Scientific Affairs. 1989. *Stewardship of the Environment.* Chicago.

Bertrand, Gerard (president, Massachusetts Audubon Society). 1990. Private communication to author.

Canby, Thomas Y. 1980. "Water—Our Most Precious Resource." *National Geographic* 158, no. 2 (August), 144–179.

Carpenter, Betsy. 1991. "In a Murky Quagmire." *U.S. News and World Report,* 3 June, pp. 45–46.

Council on Environmental Quality and U.S. Department of State. 1981. *Global 2000 Report to the President.* Washington, D.C.

Council on Environmental Quality. 1989. *Environmental Trends.* Washington, D.C.: Executive Office of the President.

EPA, National Advisory Council on Environmental Policy and Technology. 1989. "Report of the Committee on Training and Education." Washington, D.C.

Fri, R. W. 1989. *Global Warming: A Policymaker's Dilemma.* Annual report, 1988. Washington, D.C.: Resources for the Future

Harrington, W. 1988. "Breaking the Deadlock on Acid Rain Control." *Resources,* no. 93 (Fall), 1–4.

Linden, Eugene. 1989. "The Death of Birth." *Time,* 2 January, pp. 32–35.

Manzer, L. E. 1990. "The CFC-Ozone Issue: Progress on the Development of Alternatives to CFCs." *Science* 249, no. 4964 (6 July), 31–35.

Morrisette, Peter M. 1990. "Negotiating Agreements on Global Change." *Resources,* no. 99 (Spring), 8–11.

National Academy of Engineering. 1989. *Technology and Environment,* ed. J. H. Ausubel and H. E. Sladovich. Washington, D.C.: National Academy Press.

O'Connor, P. A., ed. 1977. *Congress and the Nation, 1973–1976.* Vol. 4. Washington, D.C.: Congressional Quarterly, Inc.

Somerville, J. 1989. "Concepts about Environmental Hazards Growing Nationwide." *American Medical News,* 4 August, p. 21.

Speth, J. G. 1989. "The Greening of Technology." *The Bridge* 19, no. 2 (Summer), 3–5.

Titus, J. G. 1989. "Impact of Warming on Sea Level." *Forum for Applied Research and Public Policy* 4, no. 4 (Winter), 31–36.

Warrick, Richard A., and Philip D. Jones. 1988. "The Greenhouse Effect: Impacts and Policies." *Forum for Applied Research and Public Policy* 3, no. 3 (Fall), 48–62.

World Resources Institute. 1990. *World Resources—1990–91: A Guide to the Global Environment.* New York: Oxford University Press.

Credits

Tables

1.2   Adapted from R. Doll and R. Peto, "The Causes of Cancer: Quantitative Estimates of Avoidable Risks of Cancer in the United States Today," *Journal of the National Cancer Institute* 66, no. 6 (June 1981), table 20, p. 1256.

2.1   Based on data in EPA, *National Air Quality and Emissions Trends Report,* Report EPA 450/4-91-003 (Research Triangle Park, N.C.: Office of Air Quality Planning and Standards, 1991).

2.2   Based on Paul Urone, "The Pollutants," in *Air Pollution*, vol. 6, ed. Arthur C. Stern, 3d ed. (New York: Harcourt Brace Jovanovich, 1986), table VIII, 24–25.

2.3   J. D. Spengler and K. Sexton, "Indoor Air Pollution: A Public Health Perspective," *Science* 221, no. 4605 (1 July 1983), table 1, p. 11. Copyright 1983 by the AAAS.

2.4   Based on ibid., table 2, p. 13. Copyright 1983 by the AAAS.

3.2   CDC, "Prevention of Leading Work-Related Diseases and Injuries," *Morbidity and Mortality Weekly Report* (21 January 1983), table 1, p. 25.

3.3, 3.4 Based on data in ACGIH, *1990–1991 Threshold Limit Values for Chemical Substances and Physical Agents and Biological Exposure Indices* (Cincinnati, 1990), pp. 11–40 and 58–65.

4.1   Sandra Postel, "Increasing Water Efficiency," in *State of the World,* ed. Linda Starke, Worldwatch Institute Report (New York: W. W. Norton, 1986), table 3–6, p. 55.

5.1   Based on data in Abram S. Benenson, ed., *Control of Communicable Diseases in Man,* 15th ed. (Washington, D.C.: American Public Health Association, 1990); Frank L. Bryan, *Foodborne Diseases and Their Control* (Atlanta: U.S. Department of Health and Human Services, Centers for Disease Control, 1980); and Norton Nelson and James L. Whittenberger, *Human Health and the Environment: Some Research Needs,* DHEW Publication NIH 77-1277 (Washington, D.C.: U.S. Government Printing Office, 1977).

Tables

5.2, 5.3   Adapted from N. H. Bean and P. M. Griffin, "Foodborne Disease Outbreaks in the United States, 1973–1987: Pathogens, Vehicles, and Trends," *Journal of Food Protection* 53, no. 9 (September 1990), table 7, p. 814; table 8, p. 815.

5.4   Abram S. Benenson, ed., *Control of Communicable Diseases in Man,* 15th ed. (Washington, D.C.: American Public Health Association, 1990), p. 171.

6.1   EPA, *RCRA Orientation Manual,* Report EPA/530-SW-86-001 (Washington, D.C., 1986), pp. II–9, III–4, and IV–3.

6.3   EPA, *Solving the Hazardous Waste Problem: EPA's RCRA Program,* Report EPA/530-SW-86-037 (Washington, D.C., 1986), p. 8.

6.4   "EPA Releases First Interim Report to Congress on Medical Waste Management in the United States," *Journal of the Air & Waste Management Association* 40, no. 9 (September 1990), table I, p. 1214.

6.5   NRC, *Regulation of the Disposal of Low-Level Radioactive Waste: A Guide to the Nuclear Regulatory Commission's 10 CFR Part 61* (Washington, D.C.: Office of Nuclear Material Safety and Safeguards, 1989), fig. 1, p. 2a.

6.6   EPA, *Low-Level Mixed Waste: A RCRA Perspective for NRC Licensees,* Report EPA/530-SW-90-057 (Washington, D.C., 1990), p. 23.

6.8   Adapted from DOE, *Integrated Data Base for 1989: Spent Fuel and Radioactive Waste Inventories, Projections, and Characteristics,* Report DOE/RW-006, revision 5 (Washington, D.C., 1989), table 0.3, p. 14.

6.9   E. Peelle and R. Ellis, "Beyond the 'Not-in-My-Backyard' Impasse," *Forum for Applied Research and Public Policy* 2, no. 3 (1987), table 1, p. 72.

7.1   Based on data in Pan American Health Organization, *Emergency Vector Control after Natural Disaster,* Scientific Publication no. 419 (Washington, D.C., 1982), p. 18.

7.2   Based on data in American Public Health Association, "Tropical Diseases Affect One-Tenth the World's Population," *Nation's Health* 20, no. 7 (July 1990), 8–9.

8.1   National Safety Council, *Accident Facts, 1990 Edition* (Chicago, 1990), p. 34.

9.1   Based on Committee on Interagency Radiation Research and Policy Coordination, *SI Metric Radiation Units* (Washington, D.C.: Executive Office of the President, 1986), pp. 1–3.

Tables

9.2   Adapted from Federal Radiation Council, *Background Material for the Development of Radiation Protection Standards*, Report no. 1 (Washington, D.C., 1960), table 2.1, p. 5.

9.3   Adapted from NCRP, *Ionizing Radiation Exposure of the Population of the United States*, Report no. 93 (Bethesda, Md., 1987), table 8.1, p. 53.

10.2   Based on data in ICRP, *Recommendations of the International Commission on Radiological Protection*, ICRP Publications 1, 9, 26 (New York: Pergamon Press, 1959, 1966, 1977); and ICRP, *1990 Recommendations of the International Commission on Radiological Protection*, ICRP Publication 60, Annals of the ICRP, vol. 21, no. 1–3 (New York: Pergamon Press, 1991).

10.3   Based on data in ICRP, *1990 Recommendations of the International Commission on Radiological Protection*, ICRP Publication 60, Annals of the ICRP, vol. 21, no. 1–3 (New York: Pergamon Press, 1991); and NCRP, *Recommendations on Limits for Exposure to Ionizing Radiation*, Report no. 91 (Bethesda, Md., 1987).

10.4, 10.5   Based on data in ICRP, *1990 Recommendations of the International Commission on Radiological Protection*, ICRP Publication 60, Annals of the ICRP, vol. 21, no. 1–3 (New York: Pergamon Press, 1991).

10.6   Based on data in ICRP, *Annual Limits on Intake of Radionuclides by Workers Based on the 1990 Recommendations*, ICRP Publication 61, Annals of the ICRP, vol. 21, no. 4 (New York: Pergamon Press, 1991).

11.2   Based on data in J. P. Corley, D. H. Denham, R. E. Jaquish, D. E. Michels, A. R. Olsen, and D. A. Waite, *A Guide for Environmental Radiological Surveillance at ERDA Installations*, Report ERDA-77-24 (Springfield, Va.: U.S. Department of Energy, National Technical Information Service, 1977); and D. W. Moeller, J. M. Selby, D. A. Waite, and J. P. Corley, "Environmental Surveillance for Nuclear Facilities," *Nuclear Safety* 19, no. 1 (January–February 1978), table 3, p. 73.

11.4   D. W. Moeller, J. M. Selby, D. A. Waite, and J. P. Corley, "Environmental Surveillance for Nuclear Facilities," *Nuclear Safety* 19, no. 1 (January–February 1978), table 2, p. 71.

12.2   Based on data in NCRP, *Carbon-14 in the Environment*, Report no. 81 (Bethesda, Md., 1985); and J. Tichler, K. Norden, and J. Congemi, *Radioactive Materials Released from Nuclear*

Tables

Power Plants: Annual Report 1987, Report NUREG/CR-2907, vol. 8 (Washington, D.C.: U.S. Nuclear Regulatory Commission, 1989).

12.3 Based on NRC, "Standards for Protection against Radiation," Code of Federal Regulations, Title 10, Part 20, app. B., table II.

13.2 Adapted from a chart provided by Pan American Health Organization, Washington, D.C.

13.4–13.6, 13.9 ICRP, *Protection of the Public in the Event of Major Radiation Accidents,* Publication 40, Annals of the ICRP, vol. 14, no. 2 (New York: Pergamon Press, 1984), tables 1 and 2, p. 8; table C1, p. 20; table C2, p. 21. Copyright 1984, Pergamon Press.

13.7 Adapted from B. Shleien, G. D. Schmidt, and R. P. Chiacchierini, *Background for Protective Action Recommendations: Accidental Radioactive Contamination of Food and Animal Feeds,* Publication FDA 82-8196 (Rockville, Md.: Bureau of Radiological Health, U.S. Department of Health and Human Services, 1982), table 17, p. 28.

13.8 Adapted from Federal Radiation Council, *Background Material for the Development of Radiation Protection Standards,* Report no. 5 (Washington, D.C., 1964), pp. 14 and 16; idem, *Background Material for the Development of Radiation Protection Standards: Protective Action Guides for Strontium-89, Strontium-90, and Cesium-137,* Report no. 7 (Washington, D.C., 1965), table 3, p. 16.

14.1 Cynthia P. Shea, "Mending the Earth's Shield," *World-Watch* 2, no. 1 (January–February 1989), table 1, p. 28.

14.2 Edward C. Wolf, "Survival of the Rarest," *World-Watch* 4, no. 2 (March–April 1991), 16.

14.3 National Academy of Engineering, *Technology and Environment,* ed. J. E. Ausubel and H. E. Sladovich (Washington, D.C.: National Academy Press, 1989), table 1, p. 5.

Figures

1.1 Wayne R. Ott, "Total Human Exposure: Basic Concepts, EPA Field Studies, and Future Research," *Journal of the Air & Waste Management Association* 40, no. 7 (July 1990), fig. 1, p. 968.

1.2 Ralph L. Kenney, "Mortality Risks Induced by Economic Expenditures," *Risk Analysis* 10, no. 1 (1990), p. 153.

2.1–2.3 EPA, *National Air Quality and Emissions Trends Report, 1988,* Report EPA-450/4-90-002 (Washington, D.C., 1990), pp. 13, 11, and 5.

Figures

2.4   Adapted from A. V. Nero, M. B. Schwehr, W. W. Nazaroff, and K. L. Revzan, "Distribution of Airborne Radon-222 Concentrations in U.S. Homes," *Science* 234, no. 4779 (21 November 1986), fig. 2, p. 995. Copyright 1986 by the AAAS.

3.2   Adapted from ACGIH, *Industrial Ventilation: A Manual of Recommended Practice,* 20th ed. (Lansing, Mich.: Committee on Industrial Ventilation, 1988), fig. VS–202, p. 5–21.

3.3   G. W. Morgan, "Laboratory Design," in *Radiation Hygiene Handbook,* ed. H. Blatz (New York: McGraw-Hill, 1959), fig. 9–1, p. 9–5.

3.4   National Institute for Occupational Safety and Health, *Occupational Safety and Health Guidance Manual for Hazardous Waste Site Activities* (Washington, D.C.: U.S. Department of Health and Human Services, 1985), fig. 8–2, p. 8–3.

3.5   Adapted from Barry S. Levy and David H. Wegman, eds., *Occupational Health: Recognizing and Preventing Work-Related Disease,* 2d ed. (Boston: Little, Brown, 1988), fig. 22–6, p. 360.

4.1   Council on Environmental Quality, *Environmental Trends* (Washington, D.C.: Executive Office of the President, 1989), p. 21.

5.1   Adapted from F. L. Bryan, *Foodborne Diseases and Their Control* (Atlanta: Centers for Disease Control, U.S. Department of Health and Human Services, 1980), fig. 4–1, p. 2.

6.1   Washington State Department of Ecology, *Solid Waste Landfill Design Manual* (Olympia, 1987), fig. 4.26.

6.2   EPA, *Low-Level Mixed Waste: A RCRA Perspective for NRC Licensees,* Report EPA/530-SW-90-057 (Washington, D.C., 1990), p. 3.

6.3   EPA staff.

6.4   Adapted from NRC, *Information Digest, 1991 Edition,* NUREG-1350, vol. 3 (Washington, D.C., 1991), fig. 25, p. 53.

6.5   Adapted from NRC, *Recommendations to the NRC for Review Criteria for Alternative Methods for Low-Level Radioactive Waste Disposal,* NUREG/CR-5041, vol. 1 (Washington, D.C., 1987), fig. 2.8.1, p. 2.8.2

6.6   DOE staff.

6.7   S. W. Long, *The Incineration of Low-Level Radioactive Waste,* Report NUREG-1393 (Washington, D.C.: U.S. Nuclear Regulatory Commission, 1990), app. A, p. 2.

7.1   "Publications for Rat Control and Prevention Programs," *Public Health Reports* 80, no. 1 (January 1970), p. 40.

Figures

8.1, 8.2   Adapted from Insurance Institute for Highway Safety, *Twenty Years of Accomplishment by the Insurance Institute for Highway Safety* (Arlington, Va., 1989), pp. 2, 21.

9.3   BEIR, *The Effects on Populations of Exposures to Low Levels of Ionizing Radiation: 1980,* Report no. III (Washington, D.C.: National Academy Press, 1980), fig. II–2, p. 23.

9.5   NCRP, *Ionizing Radiation Exposure of the Population of the United States,* Report no. 93 (Bethesda, Md., 1987), fig. 8.1, p. 55.

9.7   NRC, *Information Digest, 1991 Edition,* NUREG-1350, vol. 3 (Washington, D.C., 1991), fig. 7, p. 17.

10.1   Based on data in Lauriston S. Taylor, "History of the International Commission on Radiological Protection (ICRP)," *Health Physics* 1, no. 2 (1959), 97–104; and ICRP, *1990 Recommendations of the International Commission on Radiological Protection,* ICRP Publication 60, Annals of the ICRP, vol. 21, no. 1–3 (New York: Pergamon Press, 1991).

10.2   Based on data in D. C. Kocher, "Review of Radiation Protection and Environmental Radiation Standards for the Public," *Nuclear Safety* 29, no. 4 (October–December 1988), 463–475.

11.1   ICRP, *Principles of Monitoring for the Radiation Protection of the Population,* Publication 43, Annals of the ICRP, vol. 15, no. 1 (Vienna: Pergamon Press, 1985), fig. 3, p. 16. Copyright 1985, Pergamon Press.

11.2, 11.3   Ibid., figs. 1 and 2, p. 8. Copyright 1985, Pergamon Press.

12.2   Based on data provided by the U.S. Council on Energy Awareness, Washington, D.C., and on data in Council on Environmental Quality, *Environmental Trends* (Washington, D.C.: Executive Office of the President, 1989), p. 15.

12.3   Provided by U.S. Council on Energy Awareness, Washington, D.C.

13.1   U.S. Atomic Energy Commission, *Radioactive Iodine in the Problem of Radiation Safety* (translated from a USSR report) (Washington, D.C., 1972).

13.2   D. W. Moeller, "A Review of Countermeasures for Radionuclide Releases," *Radiation Protection Management* 3, no. 5 (October 1986), fig. 1, p. 72.

13.3   Federal Radiation Council, *Background for the Development of Radiation Protection Standards: Protective Action Guides for Strontium-89, Strontium-90, and Cesium-137,* Report no. 7 (Washington, D.C., 1965), fig. 2, p. 15.

Index